Voice Disorders in Fibromyalgia

Abdul-latif Hamdan
Robert Thayer Sataloff • Mary J. Hawkshaw

Voice Disorders in Fibromyalgia

Springer

Abdul-latif Hamdan
Department of Otolaryngology –
Head and Neck Surgery
American University of Beirut
Medical Center
Beirut, Lebanon

Mary J. Hawkshaw
Department of Otolaryngology –
Head and Neck Surgery
Drexel University College of Medicine
Philadelphia, PA, USA

Robert Thayer Sataloff
Department of Otolaryngology –
Head and Neck Surgery
Drexel University College of Medicine
Philadelphia, PA, USA

ISBN 978-3-031-97750-3 ISBN 978-3-031-97751-0 (eBook)
https://doi.org/10.1007/978-3-031-97751-0

This Springer imprint is published by the registered company Springer Nature Switzerland AG
The registered company address is: Gewerbestrasse 11, 6330 Cham, Switzerland

Preface

Fibromyalgia (FM) is a common condition affecting at least 2% of the population in the United States, amounting to at least five million people. It is more common among women than men. The average age at onset is 35–45 years, but it can occur in people from 25 to 55 years of age. Generalized pain involving the musculoskeletal system is the most prominent symptom, but FM can also involve other body systems as well. FM causes cognitive impairment, mood alterations, imbalance, generalized fatigue, dyspepsia, and other symptoms. FM and its treatments can affect the voice adversely. Dysphonia associated with FM has received relatively little attention from clinicians and researchers. This book is intended to summarize FM for the convenience of laryngologists and other voice care professionals, highlighting what is known and what is suspected about its effects on voice. This book is also intended to crystallize voice consequences and its treatments for rheumatologists, orthopedists, and others involved commonly in the care of patients with FM, but whom might not be cognizant of the presence and importance of voice disturbance in the FM population.

Chapter 1 provides an overview of the problem of FM and dysphonia. Chapter 2 reviews the anatomy and physiology of phonation and should serve as a useful review for otolaryngologists and particularly as a helpful reference for other healthcare providers. Chapter 3 provides an overview of the complex history, physical examination, and testing that should be performed for patients with voice disorders, including selected tests that should be added in patients with diagnosed or suspected FM. Chapter 4 summarizes information that is known well to physicians and specialists who treat FM patients commonly but less well to voice specialists. It reviews the clinical presentation, pathophysiology, and diagnosis of Fibromyalgia syndrome. Chapter 5 discusses the prevalence of voice disorders in FM, although voice disorders are discussed specifically in each targeted chapter. Chapter 6 reviews respiratory dysfunction which is common in Fibromyalgia and highlights the important consequences of impairment of the "power source" of the voice, a problem that can lead not only to voice weakness and fatigue but also to compensatory hyperfunction of neck muscles and related vocal fold trauma and masses. Chapter 7 discusses gastrointestinal disorders in Fibromyalgia. They are common in FM, and they are also common in voice patients, particularly laryngopharyngeal reflux which may be aggravated by FM. Chapter 8 reviews the association of FM with rheumatologic diseases. Many rheumatologic conditions are associated with dysphonia, and the increased prevalence of rheumatologic problems in FM patients is associated with an increased prevalence of voice problems. Pain and central sensitization are discussed in Chap. 9, along with their voice consequences. Fibromyalgia is also associated routinely with reduced muscle strength. The problem and its causes are reviewed in Chap. 10, along with expected voice consequences. Autonomic nervous system dysfunction is also common in Fibromyalgia and is well known to be associated with dysphonia, as reviewed in Chap. 11. Chapter 12 highlights the extremely common problem of sleep disorders in people with FM. Various aspects of sleep impairment and its treatments are well established as causes of dysphonia. Chapter 13 provides insights into depression and chronic fatigue syndrome which are more common in FM patients than in the general population. Those conditions are also known to cause voice problems, as discussed in the chapter. Fibromyalgia is also associated very commonly with obesity and suboptimal dietary habits. The effects of obesity on the voice as discussed in Chap. 14 are so important that an entire book has been written on the subject [1], and FM-associated obesity causes the same voice problems as does obesity from other causes. As stressed in Chap. 15, dysphonia can be caused not only by FM but also by treatment of FM, particularly pharmacologic treatment. This chapter reviews the medications used commonly for FM and provides a table summarizing their voice-related side effects. This should be helpful for physicians trying to diagnose voice problems in patients being treated for FM, as well as for health care professionals treating FM, especially in professional voice users in whom it is helpful to tailor treatment to minimize laryngologic side effects. Chapter 16 summarizes the knowledge and gaps identified in the previous chapters and highlights the importance of future research.

This is the first book on this important topic. We hope that our readers find it not only informative and useful but also inspirational. A great deal of additional research is needed to understand fully the relationship between FM and dysphonia and to provide patients with optimal treatment.

Reference

1. Hamdan AL, Sataloff RT, Hawkshaw MJ. Obesity and voice. San Diego: Plural Publishing; 2020.

Beirut, Lebanon — Abdul Latif Hamdan
Philadelphia, PA, USA — Robert Thayer Sataloff
Philadelphia, PA, USA — Mary J. Hawkshaw

Contents

Introduction

1

Abdul-latif Hamdan, Robert Thayer Sataloff,
and Mary J. Hawkshaw

Fibromyalgia (FM) is a chronic disorder that affects millions of people yearly. It is estimated that 2–5% of the general population suffer from this syndrome, with a female to male ratio ranging from 2:1 to 6:1. Familial aggregation has been described with an increased risk of having FMS in case of a positive family history [1, 2]. Fibromyalgia is characterized by persistent diffuse pain and tenderness at multiple sites of the musculoskeletal system. The widespread body aches often are associated with chronic fatigue, sleep disturbance, insomnia, cognitive disability, mood alteration, anxiety, depression, dyspnea and gastro-intestinal symptoms among others. The pathophysiology of FM is complex. Many theories have been suggested with no clear consensus on the etiology of this syndrome. These include central sensitization with impairment in the descending inhibitory pathways, abnormalities in muscle tissue metabolism, and dysfunction in the autoimmune system. Given that the larynx is a musculoskeletal structure, it is subject to the systemic manifestation of this syndrome. Dysfunction in the respiratory muscles jeopardizes the power source of the phonatory system [3, 4], and decreased laryngeal muscle strength/endurance can lead to impairment in voice production [5–7]. Similarly, alteration in pain processing and central sensitization may increase the risk of functional voice disorders [8].

Patients with FM suffer from many co-morbidities, the frequency and list of which is increasing with time in view of our better understanding of the disease and improved accessibility to healthcare services. These include mental disorders such as anxiety/depression, rheumatologic diseases such as rheumatoid arthritis, gastro-intestinal diseases such as irritable bowel syndrome and gastro-esophageal reflux disease, hypothyroidism, autonomic nervous system dysfunction and dysregulation in the respiratory system among others. All these co-morbidities have adverse effects on the phonatory system. Psychiatric illnesses are associated with alteration in pitch, loudness and changes in the prosodic features of speech [9, 10]. Rheumatologic diseases affect the di-arthrodial joints of the laryngeal framework leading to impairment in the mobility of the vocal folds [11]. The decrease in chest

A.-l. Hamdan et al., *Voice Disorders in Fibromyalgia*,
https://doi.org/10.1007/978-3-031-97751-0_1

wall compliance and reduced maximal expiratory pressure in patients with FM may jeopardize breath support and control, which are of paramount importance in professional voice users [12]. Almost one out of five patients with FM suffers from gastrointestinal disturbances including reflux disease, a known risk factor for structural and functional voice disorders. Obesity as result of inactivity and deconditioning is also a common comorbidity present in 20% of patients with FM. Patients with a high body mass index have been shown to exhibit different voice characteristics compared with those with a low body mass index. Several mechanisms have been suggested among which are changes in vocal tract morphology, reduced breathing capacity, and alteration in sex hormones.

This book presents a review of the literature on the prevalence of voice disorders in FM with a thorough deliberation on the pathophysiology of dysphonia in affected patients, namely the adverse effects of muscle dysfunction and decrease in respiratory capacity on voice. The authors also review the laryngeal manifestation of the numerous comorbidities associated with FM, such as chronic fatigue syndrome, gastro-esophageal reflux disease, obesity, sleep apnea, and autonomic nervous system dysfunction and their impact on phonation. Treatment-induced changes in voice quality are also highlighted in the context of this syndrome and future research projects on the link between FM and phonation are highlighted.

References

1. Arnold LM, Hudson JI, Hess EV, Ware AE, Fritz DA, Auchenbach MB, Starck LO, Keck PE Jr. Family study of fibromyalgia. Arthritis Rheum. 2004;50(3):944–52.
2. Chakrabarty S, Zoorob R. Fibromyalgia. Am Fam Physician. 2007;76(2):247–54.
3. Traser L, Burk F, Özen AC, Burdumy M, Bock M, Blaser D, Richter B, Echternach M. Respiratory kinematics and the regulation of subglottic pressure for phonation of pitch jumps—a dynamic MRI study. PLoS One. 2020;15(12):e0244539.
4. Traser L, Özen AC, Burk F, Burdumy M, Bock M, Richter B, Echternach M. Respiratory dynamics in phonation and breathing-a real-time MRI study. Respir Physiol Neurobiol. 2017;236:69–7.
5. Hamdan AL, Hosri J, Yammine Y, Ghzayel L, Hadi J, Moussawi MA, Romanos M, Nader N, Uthman I. Voice disorders in patients with fibromyalgia: case series and review of the literature. J Voice. 2024; https://doi.org/10.1016/j.jvoice.2024.06.027.
6. Hamdan AL, Alam E, Feghali PAR, Fadel C, Jabbour C, Ghanem A. Risk of fibromyalgia in patients with primary muscle tension dysphonia: a possible local manifestation of a musculoskeletal systemic disorder. J Laryngol Otol. 2024;138(3):341–4.
7. Gurbuzler L, Inanir A, Yelken K, Koc S, Eyibilen A, Uysal IO. Voice disorder in patients with fibromyalgia. Auris Nasus Larynx. 2013;40(6):554–7.
8. Piersiala K, Akst LM, Hillel AT, Best SR. Chronic pain syndromes and their laryngeal manifestations. JAMA Otolaryngol Head Neck Surg. 2020;146(6):543–9.
9. Silva WJ, Lopes L, Galdino MK, Almeida AA. Voice acoustic parameters as predictors of depression. J Voice. 2024;38(1):77–85.

10. Taguchi T, Tachikawa H, Nemoto K, Suzuki M, Nagano T, Tachibana R, Nishimura M, Arai T. Major depressive disorder discrimination using vocal acoustic features. J Affect Disord. 2018;225:214–20.
11. Voulgari PV, Papazisi D, Bai M, Zagorianakou P, Assimakopoulos D, Drosos AA. Laryngeal involvement in rheumatoid arthritis. Rheumatol Int. 2005;25:321–5.
12. Ozgocmen S, Cimen OB, Ardicoglu O. Relationship between chest expansion and respiratory muscle strength in patients with primary fibromyalgia. Clin Rheumatol. 2002;21:19–22.

Anatomy and Physiology of the Voice

2

Abdul-latif Hamdan, Robert Thayer Sataloff,
and Mary J. Hawkshaw

To treat voice patients knowledgeably and responsibly, health care providers must understand the medical aspects of voice disorders and their treatment. This requires core knowledge of the anatomy and physiology of phonation. The human voice consists of much more than simply the vocal folds, popularly known as the vocal cords. State-of-the-art voice diagnosis, nonsurgical therapy, and voice surgery depend on understanding the complex workings of the vocal tract. Physicians and other health care professionals specializing in the care of voice patients, especially voice professionals, should be familiar with at least the basics of the latest concepts in voice function. The physiology of phonation is much more complex than this brief chapter might suggest, and readers interested in acquiring more than a clinically essential introduction are encouraged to consult other literature [1].

Anatomy

The larynx is essential to normal voice production, but the anatomy of the voice is not limited to the larynx. The vocal mechanism includes the abdominal and back musculature, rib cage, lungs, pharynx, oral cavity, and nose, among other structures. Each component performs an important function in voice production, although it is possible to produce voice even without a larynx—for example, in patients who have undergone laryngectomy. In addition, virtually all parts of the body play some role in voice production and may be responsible for voice dysfunction. Even something as remote as a sprained ankle may alter posture, thereby impairing abdominal, back, and thoracic muscle function and resulting in vocal inefficiency, weakness, and hoarseness.

A.-l. Hamdan et al., *Voice Disorders in Fibromyalgia*,
https://doi.org/10.1007/978-3-031-97751-0_2

The larynx is composed of four basic anatomic units: skeleton, intrinsic muscles, extrinsic muscles, and mucosa. The most important components of the laryngeal skeleton are the thyroid cartilage, cricoid cartilage, and two arytenoid cartilages (Fig. 2.1). Intrinsic muscles of the larynx are connected to these cartilages (Fig. 2.2). One of the intrinsic muscles, the *thyroarytenoid muscle* (its medial belly also is known as the vocalis muscle), extends on each side from the vocal process of the arytenoid cartilage to the inside of the thyroid cartilage just below and behind the thyroid prominence ("Adam's apple"), forming the body of the vocal folds. The vocal folds act as the *oscillator* or *voice source* of the vocal tract. The space between the vocal folds is called the *glottis* and is used as an anatomic reference point. The intrinsic muscles alter the position, shape, and tension of the vocal folds, bringing them together (adduction), moving them apart (abduction), or stretching them by increasing longitudinal tension (Fig. 2.3). They are able to do so because the laryngeal cartilages are connected by soft attachments that allow changes in their relative angles and distances, thereby permitting alteration in the shape and tension of the tissues suspended between them. The arytenoid cartilages on their eliptoid cricoarytenoid joints are capable of motion in multiple planes, permitting complex vocal fold motion and alteration in the shape of the vocal fold edge associated with intrinsic muscle action (Fig. 2.4). All but one of the muscles on each side of the larynx are innervated by one of the two *recurrent laryngeal nerves*. Because this nerve runs in a long course (especially on the left) from the neck down into the chest and then back up to the larynx (hence, the name "recurrent"), it is injured easily by trauma, neck surgery, and chest surgery. Injury may result in vocal fold paresis or paralysis. The remaining muscle (*cricothyroid muscle*) is innervated by the superior laryngeal nerve on each side, which is especially susceptible to viral and traumatic injury. It causes changes in longitudinal tension that are important in voice projection and pitch control. The "false vocal folds" are located above the vocal folds, and unlike the true vocal folds, usually do not make contact during normal speaking or singing [1]. The neuroanatomy and neurophysiology of phonation are extremely complicated, and only partially understood. As the new field of neurolaryngology advances, a more thorough understanding of the subject is becoming increasingly important to clinicians. Readers interested in acquiring a deeper, scientific understanding of neurolaryngology are encouraged to consult other literature [2] and the publications cited therein.

Because the attachments of the laryngeal cartilages are flexible, the positions of the cartilages with respect to each other change when the laryngeal skeleton is elevated or lowered. Such changes in vertical height are controlled by the extrinsic laryngeal muscles, the strap muscles of the neck. When the angles and distances between cartilages change because of this accordion-like effect, the resting length of the intrinsic muscle changes. Such large adjustments in intrinsic muscle condition interfere with fine control of smooth vocal quality. Classically trained singers generally are taught to use the extrinsic muscles to maintain the laryngeal skeleton at a relatively constant height regardless of pitch. That is, they learn to

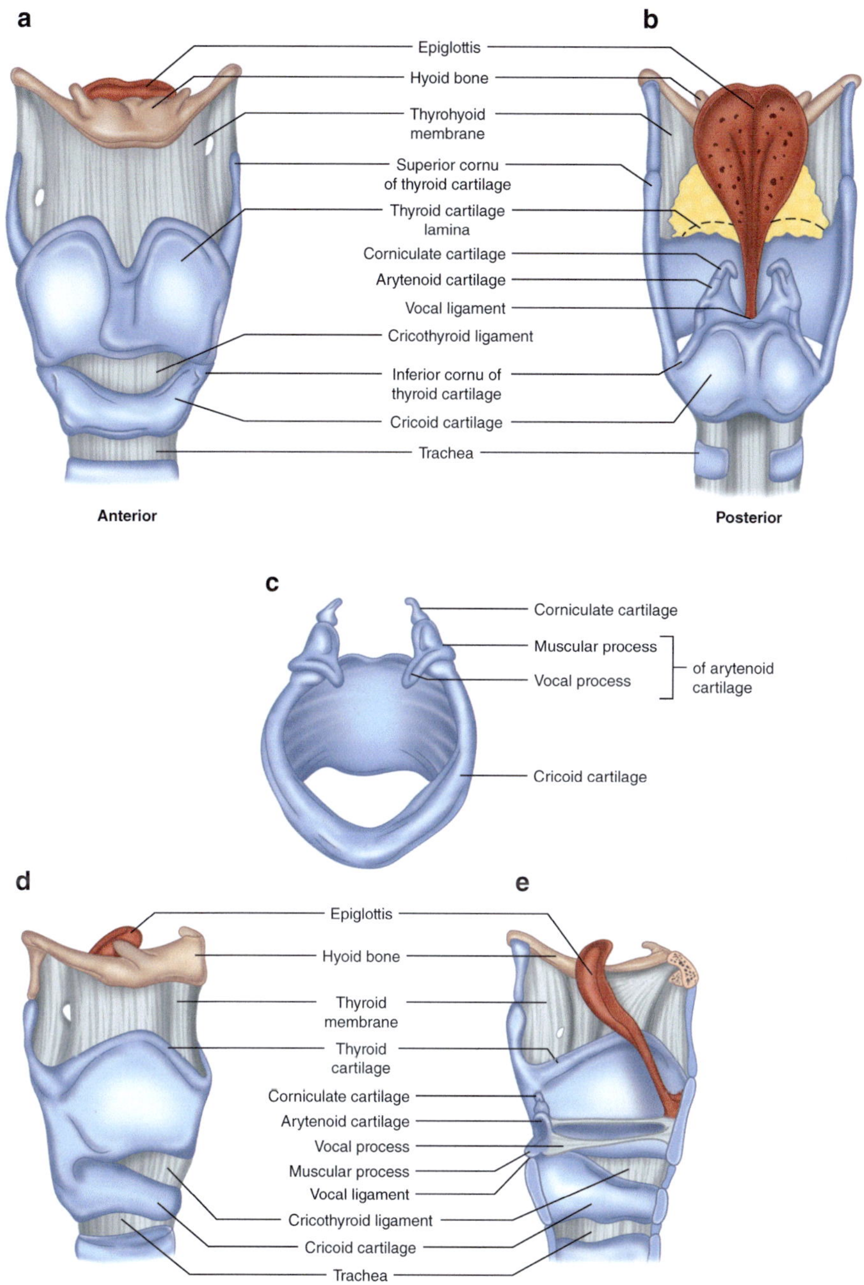

Fig. 2.1 Cartilages of the larynx in anterior (**a**), posterior (**b**), isolated cricoid and bilateral arytenoid cartilages (**c**), right lateral external (**d**), and right lateral internal (**e**) views

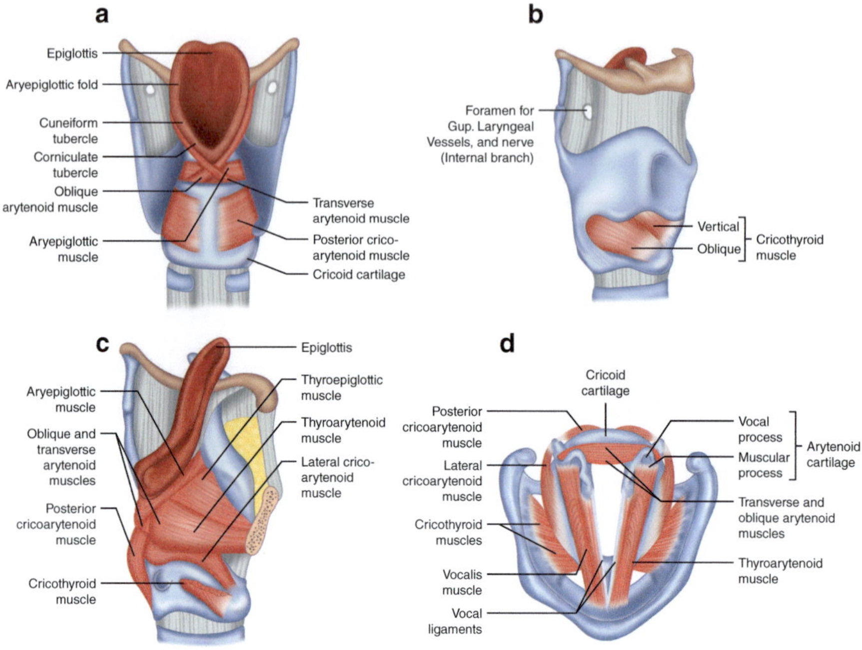

Fig. 2.2 Intrinsic muscles of the larynx from posterior (**a**), anterior (**b**), right internal (**c**), and above (**d**)

avoid the natural tendency of the larynx to rise with ascending pitch and fall with descending pitch, thereby enhancing unity of sound quality throughout the vocal range through effects on both resting muscle condition and supraglottic vocal tract posture.

The soft tissues lining the larynx are much more complex than originally thought. The mucosa forms the thin, lubricated surface of the vocal folds, which makes contact when the two vocal folds are approximated. Laryngeal mucosa might look superficially like the mucosa which lines the inside of the mouth, but it is not. Throughout most of the larynx, there are goblet cells and pseudo-stratified ciliated columnar epithelial cells designed for producing and handling mucous secretions, similar to mucosal surfaces found throughout the respiratory tract. However, the mucosa overlying the vocal folds is different. First, it is stratified squamous epithelium, which is better suited to withstand the trauma of vocal fold contact. Second, the vocal fold is not simply muscle covered with mucosa. Rather, it consists of five layers as described by Hirano [3]. Mechanically, the vocal fold structures act more like three layers consisting of the *cover* (epithelium layer and superficial layer of the lamina propria), *transition* (intermediate and deep layers of the lamina propria), and *body* (the vocalis muscle).

The *supraglottic vocal tract* includes the pharynx, tongue, palate, oral cavity, nose, and other structures. Together, they act as a *resonator* and are largely

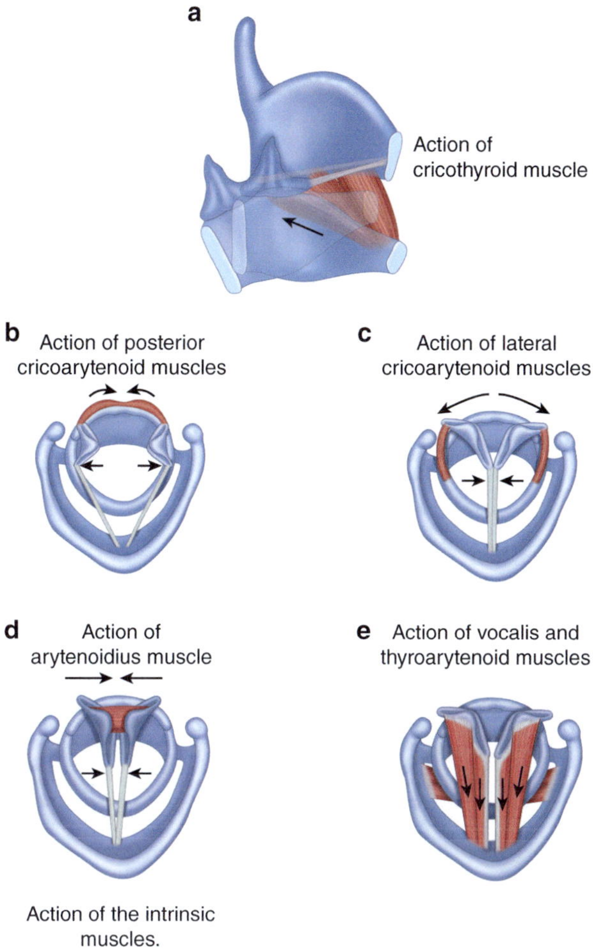

Fig. 2.3 Action of the intrinsic muscles including cricothyroid (**a**), posterior cricoarytenoid (**b**), lateral cricoarytenoid (**c**), arytenoideus (interarytenoid) (**d**), and thyroarytenoid (**e**)

responsible for vocal quality or timbre and the perceived character of all phonated sounds. The vocal folds themselves produce only a "buzzing" sound. During the course of vocal training for singing, acting, or healthy speaking, changes occur not only in the larynx, but also in the muscle motion, control, and shape of the supraglottic vocal tract, and in aerobic, pulmonary, and bodily muscle function.

The *infraglottic vocal tract* (all anatomical structures below the glottis) serves as the *power source* for the voice. Singers and actors often refer to the entire power source complex as their "support" or "diaphragm." The anatomy of support for phonation is especially complicated and not completely understood. Yet, it is quite important because deficiencies in support frequently are responsible for voice dysfunction.

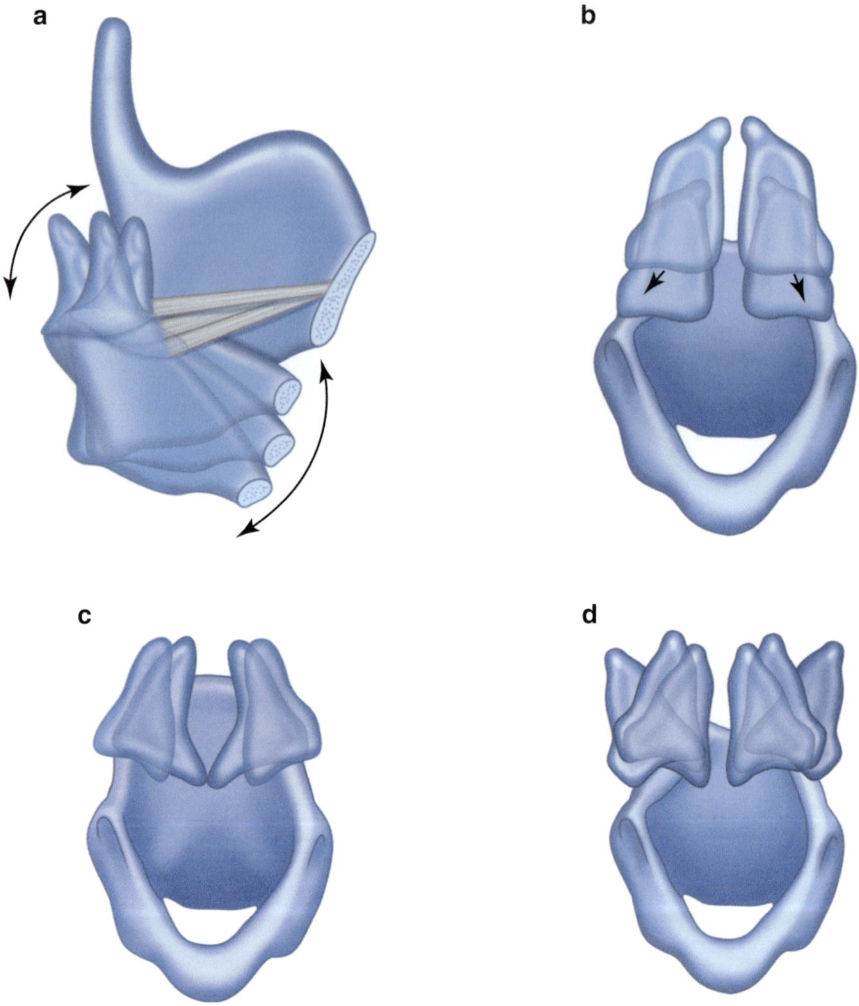

Fig. 2.4 Complex arytenoid motion including cricothyroid joint (**a**), cricoarytenoid joint gliding (**b**), rotating (**c**), and rocking (**d**)

The purpose of the support mechanism is to generate a force that directs a controlled airstream between the vocal folds. Active respiratory muscles work in concert with passive forces. The principal muscles of inspiration are the diaphragm (a dome-shaped muscle that extends along the bottom of the rib cage) and the external intercostal muscles (located between the ribs). During quiet respiration, expiration is largely passive. The lungs and rib cage generate passive expiratory forces under many common circumstances such as after a full breath.

Many of the muscles used for active expiration also are employed in "support" for phonation. Muscles of active expiration either raise the intra-abdominal pressure, forcing the diaphragm upward, or lower the ribs or sternum to decrease the dimensions of the thorax, or both, thereby compressing air in the chest. The primary muscles of expiration are "the abdominal muscles," but internal intercostals and other chest and back muscles also are involved. Trauma or surgery that alters the structure or function of these muscles or ribs undermines the power source of the voice, as do diseases, such as asthma, that impair expiration. Deficiencies in the support mechanism often result in compensatory efforts that utilize the laryngeal muscles, which are not designed for power functions. Such behavior can result in impaired voice quality, rapid fatigue, pain, and even structural pathology such as vocal fold nodules. Current expert treatment for such vocal problems focuses on correction of the underlying malfunction rather than surgery whenever possible.

Physiology

The physiology of voice production is extremely complex. Volitional production of voice begins in the cerebral cortex (Fig. 2.5).

The command for vocalization involves complex interactions among brain centers for speech, as well as other areas. For singing, speech directives must be integrated with information from the centers for musical and artistic expression, which are discussed elsewhere [1]. The "idea" of the planned vocalization is conveyed to the precentral gyrus in the motor cortex, which transmits another set of instructions to the motor nuclei in the brainstem and spinal cord. These areas send out the complicated messages necessary for coordinated activity of the larynx, thoracic and abdominal musculature lungs, and vocal tract articulators, among other structures. Additional refinement of motor activity is provided by the extrapyramidal and autonomic nervous systems. These impulses combine to produce a sound that is transmitted not only to the ears of the listener, but also to those of the speaker or singer. Auditory feedback is transmitted from the ear through the brainstem to the cerebral cortex, and adjustments are made within milliseconds that permit the vocalist to match the sound produced with the sound intended, integrating the acoustic properties of the performance environment. Tactile feedback from throat and other muscles involved in phonation also is believed to help in fine tuning vocal output, although the mechanism and role of tactile feedback are not understood fully. Many trained singers and speakers cultivate the ability to use tactile feedback effectively because of expected interference with auditory feedback data from ancillary sound such as an orchestra or band.

Phonation, the production of sound, requires interaction among the power source, oscillator, and resonator. The voice may be compared to a brass instrument such as a trumpet. Power is generated by the chest, abdominal, and back musculature and a high-pressure air stream is produced. The trumpeter's lips open and close against the mouthpiece producing a "buzz" similar to the sound produced by vocal folds when they come together and move apart (oscillate) during phonation. This sound then passes through the trumpet, which has acoustic resonance characteristics that shape the sound we associate with trumpet music. If a trumpet mouthpiece is placed on a French horn, the sound we hear will sound like a French horn, not a trumpet.

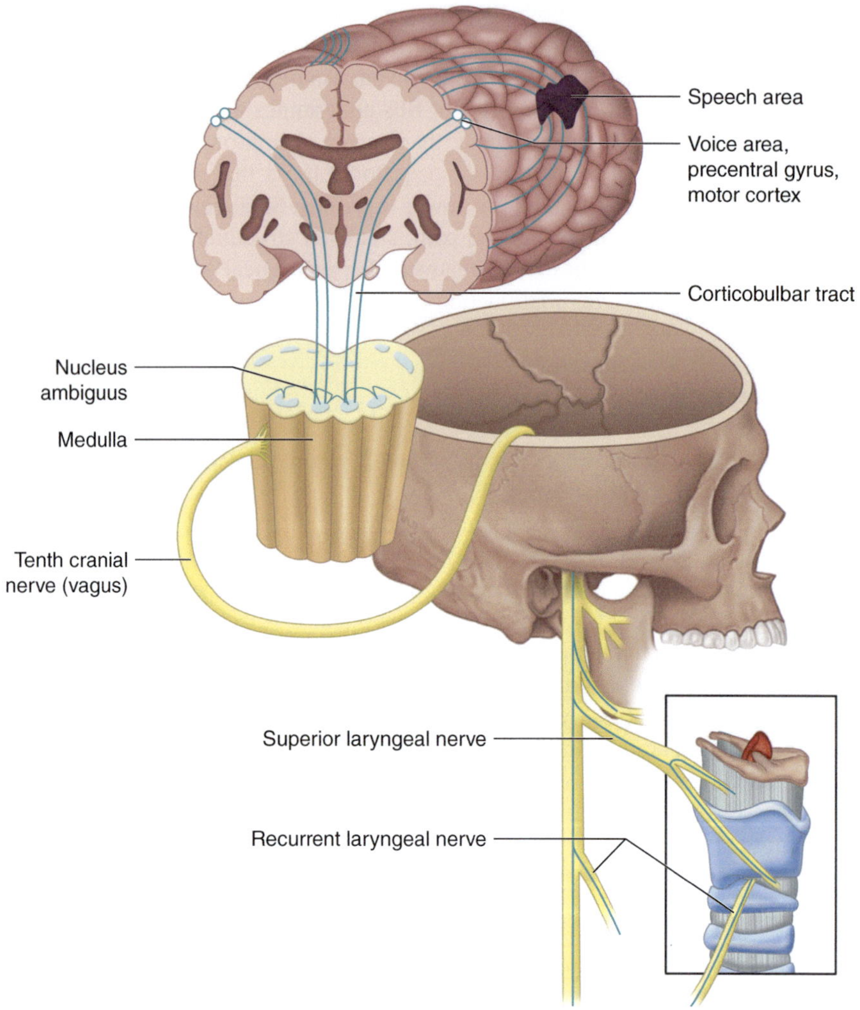

Fig. 2.5 Simplified summary of pathway for volitional phonation

Quality characteristics are dependent upon the resonator more than on the oscillatory source. The non-mouthpiece portions of a brass instrument are analogous to the supraglottic vocal tract.

During phonation, the infraglottic musculature must make rapid, complex adjustments because the resistance changes almost continuously as the glottis closes, opens, and changes shape. At the beginning of each phonatory cycle, the vocal folds are approximated, and the glottis is obliterated. This permits infraglottic air pressure to build, typically to a level of about 7 cm of water for conversational speech. At that point, the vocal folds are convergent (Fig. 2.6a). Because the vocal folds are closed, there is no airflow. The subglottic pressure then pushes the vocal folds progressively

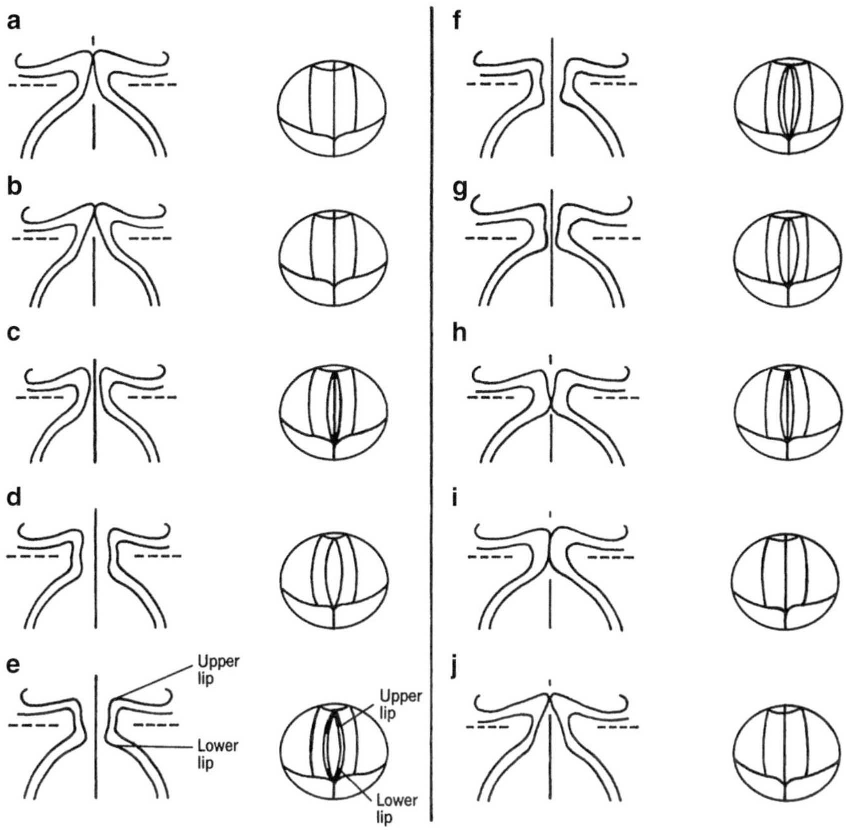

Fig. 2.6 Frontal view (left) and view from above (right) illustrating the normal pattern of vocal fold vibration. The vocal folds close and open from the inferior aspect of the vibratory margin upward, and from posterior to anterior

farther apart from the bottom up and from the back forward (Fig. 2.6b) until a space develops (Fig. 2.6c, d) and air begins to flow. Bernoulli force created by the air passing between the vocal folds combines with the mechanical properties of the folds to begin closing the lower portion of the vocal folds almost immediately (Fig. 2.6e–h) even while the upper edges are still separating. The principles and mathematics of Bernoulli force are complex. It is a flow effect more easily understood by familiar examples such as the sensation of pull exerted on a vehicle when passed by a truck at high speed or the inward motion of a shower curtain when the water flows past it.

The upper portion of the vocal folds has elastic properties that also tend to make the vocal folds snap back to the midline. This force becomes more dominant as the upper edges are stretched and the opposing force of the air stream diminishes because of approximation of the lower edges of the vocal folds. The upper portions of the vocal folds are then returned to the midline (Fig. 2.6i), completing the glottic cycle. Subglottal pressure then builds again (Fig. 2.6j), and the events repeat. Thus, there is a vertical phase difference. That is, the lower portion of the vocal folds begins to open and close before the upper portion. The rippling displacement of the vocal fold cover produces a mucosal wave that can be examined clinically under stroboscopic light. If this complex motion is impaired, hoarseness or other changes in voice quality may cause the patient to seek medical evaluation. The frequency of vibration (number of cycles of openings and closings per second, measured in hertz [Hz]) is dependent on the air pressure and mechanical properties of the vocal folds, which are regulated in part by the laryngeal muscles. Pitch is the perceptual correlate of frequency. Under most circumstances, as the vocal folds are thinned and stretched and air pressure is increased, the frequency of air pulse emissions increases, and pitch goes up. The myoelastic-aerodynamic mechanism of phonation reveals that the vocal folds emit pulses of air, rather than vibrating like strings.

The sound produced by the oscillating vocal folds, called the voice source signal, is a complex tone containing a fundamental frequency and many overtones, or higher harmonic partials. The amplitude of the partials decreases uniformly at approximately 12 dB/octave. Interestingly, the acoustic spectrum of the voice source is about the same in ordinary speakers as it is in trained singers and speakers. Voice quality differences in voice professionals occur as the voice source signal passes through their supraglottic vocal tract resonator system (Fig. 2.7).

The pharynx, oral cavity, and nasal cavity act as a series of infinitely variable interconnected resonators, which are more complex than that in our trumpet example or other single resonators. As with other resonators, some frequencies are attenuated, others are enhanced. Enhanced frequencies are radiated with higher relative amplitudes or intensities. Sundberg [4] showed long ago that the vocal tract has four or five important resonance frequencies called *formants* and summarized his early findings in a book that has become a classic. The presence of formants alters the uniformly sloping voice source spectrum and creates peaks at formant frequencies. These alterations of the voice source spectral envelope are responsible for distinguishable sounds of speech and song. Formant frequencies are determined by vocal tract shape, which can be altered by the laryngeal, pharyngeal, and oral cavity musculature. Overall vocal tract length and shape are individually fixed and determined by age and sex (females and children have shorter vocal tracts and formant frequencies that are higher than males). Voice training includes conscious physical mastery of the adjustment of vocal tract shape.

Although the formants differ for different vowels, one resonant frequency has received particular attention and is known as the "singer's formant." This formant occurs in the vicinity of 2300 to 3200 Hz for all vowel spectra and appears to be responsible for the "ring" in a singer's or trained speaker's ("speaker's formant") voice. The ability to hear a trained voice clearly even over a loud choir or orchestra is dependent primarily on the presence of the singer's formant [1]. Interestingly, there is little or no significant difference in maximum vocal intensity between trained and untrained singers. The singer's formant also contributes substantially to the differences in fach (voice classification) among voice categories, occurring in basses at about 2400 Hz, baritones at 2600 Hz, tenors at 2800 Hz, mezzo-sopranos

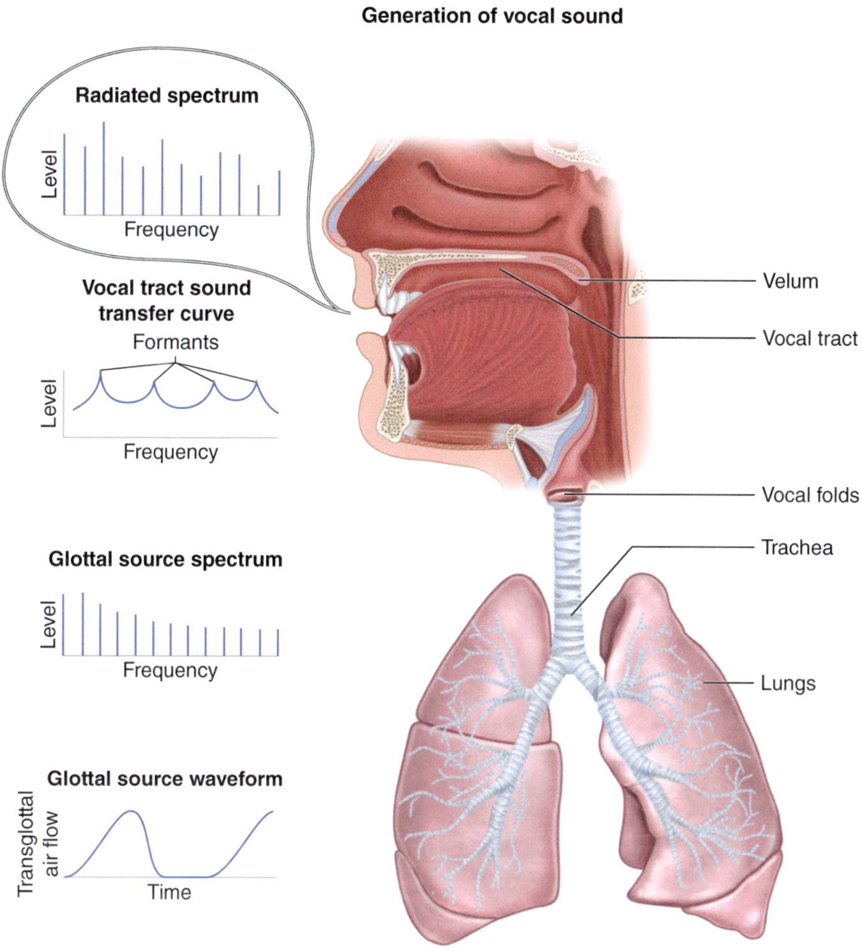

Fig. 2.7 Determinants of the spectrum of a vowel (oral-output signal)

at 2900 Hz, and sopranos at 3200 Hz. It is frequently much less prominent in high soprano singing [1].

The mechanisms that control two vocal characteristics are particularly important: fundamental frequency and intensity. Fundamental frequency, which corresponds to pitch, can be altered by changing either air pressure or the mechanical properties of the vocal folds, although the latter is more efficient under most conditions. When the cricothyroid muscle contracts, it makes the thyroid cartilage pivot on the cricothyroid cartilage and increases the distance between the thyroid and arytenoid cartilages, thus stretching the vocal folds. This increases the surface area exposed to subglottal pressure and makes the air pressure more effective in opening the glottis. In addition, stretching of elastic fibers of the vocal fold makes them more efficient at snapping back together. Hence, the cycles shorten and repeat more frequently, and the fundamental frequency (and pitch) rise. Other muscles, including the thyroarytenoid, also contribute [1]. Raising the pressure of the air stream also tends to increase fundamental frequency, a phenomenon for which singers must learn to compensate. Otherwise, their pitch would go up whenever they tried to sing more loudly.

Voice intensity corresponds to loudness and depends on the degree to which the glottal wave motion excites the air molecules in the vocal tract. Raising the air pressure creates greater amplitude of vocal fold oscillation and therefore increases vocal intensity. However, actually it is not the oscillation of the vocal fold, but rather the sudden cessation of airflow that is responsible for initiating an acoustic signal in the vocal tract and controlling intensity. This is similar to the mechanism of acoustic signal that results from buzzing lips. In the larynx, the sharper the cutoff of air flow, the more intense the sound [1]. In the evaluation of voice disorders, an individual's ability to optimize adjustments of air pressure and glottal resistance is assessed. When high subglottic pressure is combined with high adductory (closing) vocal fold force, glottal airflow and the amplitude of the voice source fundamental frequency are low. This is called *pressed phonation* and can be measured clinically through a technique known as flow glottography. Flow glottogram wave amplitude indicates the type of phonation being used, and the slope (closing rate) provides information about the sound pressure level or loudness. If adductory forces are so weak that the vocal folds do not make contact, the vocal folds become inefficient at resisting air leakage, and the voice source fundamental frequency is low. This is known as *breathy phonation*. *Flow phonation* is characterized by lower subglottic pressure and lower adductory force. These conditions increase the dominance of the fundamental frequency of the voice source in the perceived sound. Sundberg showed that the amplitude of the fundamental frequency can be increased by 15 dB or more when the subject changes from pressed phonation to flow phonation [4]. If a patient habitually uses pressed phonation, considerable effort will be required to achieve loud voicing. The muscle patterns and force that are used to compensate for this laryngeal inefficiency may cause vocal fold damage. Such voice behavior (i.e., pressed voice) can result from laryngeal structural problems, voice technique, psychological abnormalities, and other causes.

Acknowledgments Modified in part from Sataloff RT. Professional Voice: The Science and Art of Clinical Care, 4th Edition. San Diego, CA: Plural Publishing; 2017, with permission.

References

1. Sataloff RT. Professional voice: The science and art of clinical care. 4th ed. San Diego: Plural Publishing; 2017.
2. Sataloff RT. Neurolaryngology. San Diego: Plural Publishing; 2017.
3. Hirano M. Phonosurgery: basic and clinical investigations. Otologia (Fukuoka). 1975;21:239–442.
4. Sundberg J. The science of the singing voice. DeKalb: Northern Illinois University Press; 1987.

3 Evaluation of Patients with Voice Disorders

Abdul-latif Hamdan, Robert Thayer Sataloff, and Mary J. Hawkshaw

Effective history taking and physical examination depend on a practical understanding of the anatomy and physiology of voice production as discussed in Chap. 2 [1–3]. Because dysfunction in virtually any body system may affect phonation, medical inquiry must be comprehensive. The current standard of care for all voice patients evolved from advances inspired by medical problems of voice professionals such as singers and actors. However, a great many other patients are voice professionals, including teachers, salespeople, attorneys, clergy, physicians, politicians, telephone receptionists, and anyone else whose ability to earn a living is impaired in the presence of voice dysfunction.

The scope of inquiry and examination for most patients is similar to that required for singers and actors, except that performing voice professionals have unique needs that require additional history and examination. Questions must be added regarding performance commitments, professional status and voice goals, the amount and nature of voice training, the performance environment, rehearsal practices, abusive habits during speech and singing, and many other matters. Such supplementary information is essential to proper treatment selection and patient counseling in singers and actors. However, analogous factors also must be taken into account for stockbrokers, factory shop foremen, elementary school teachers, homemakers with several noisy children, and many others. Physicians familiar with the management of these challenging patients are well equipped to evaluate all patients with voice complaints. Details of the history, physical examination and work-up are beyond the scope of this summary chapter and may be found elsewhere [1].

A.-l. Hamdan et al., *Voice Disorders in Fibromyalgia*, https://doi.org/10.1007/978-3-031-97751-0_3

Patient History

Obtaining extensive historical background information is necessary for thorough evaluation of the voice patient, and it should be obtained through questions and may be supplemented with a history questionnaire [1]. Readers may consult other literature for a more complete discussion of each question posed in the history [1].

How Old Are You?

All components of voice production are subject to normal aging. Abdominal and general muscular tone frequently decrease, lungs lose elasticity, the thorax loses distensibility, the mucosa of the vocal tract atrophies, mucous secretions change character and quantity, nerve endings are reduced in number, and psychoneurologic functions change. Moreover, the larynx itself loses muscle tone and bulk and may show depletion of submucosal ground substance in the vocal folds. The laryngeal cartilages ossify, and the joints may become arthritic and stiff. Hormonal influence is altered. Vocal range, intensity, and quality all may be modified. Vocal fold atrophy may be the most striking alteration. The clinical effects of aging seem more pronounced in female singers, although vocal fold histologic changes may be more prominent in males. Excellent male singers occasionally extend their careers into their 70s or beyond [4, 5]. However, some degree of breathiness, decreased range, and other evidence of aging should be expected in elderly voices. Nevertheless, many of the changes we typically associate with elderly singers (wobble, flat pitch) are due to lack of conditioning, rather than inevitable changes of biological aging. These aesthetically undesirable concomitants of aging can often be reversed.

What Is Your Voice Problem?

Careful questioning as to the onset of vocal problems is needed to separate acute from chronic dysfunction. Often an upper respiratory tract infection will send a patient to the physician's office, but penetrating inquiry, especially in singers and actors, may reveal a chronic voice problem that is the patient's real concern.

The specific nature of the vocal complaint can provide a great deal of information. Just as dizzy patients rarely walk into the physician's office complaining of "rotary vertigo," voice patients may be unable to articulate their symptoms without guidance. They may use the term *hoarseness* to describe a variety of conditions that the physician must separate. Hoarseness is a coarse or scratchy sound that is most often associated with abnormalities of the leading edge of the vocal folds such as laryngitis or mass lesions. Breathiness is a vocal quality characterized by excessive loss of air during vocalization. In some cases, it is due to improper technique.

However, any condition that prevents full approximation of the vocal folds can be responsible. Possible causes include vocal fold paralysis, a mass lesion separating the leading edges of the vocal folds, arthritis of the cricoarytenoid joint, arytenoid dislocation, scarring of the vibratory margin, senile vocal fold atrophy (presbyphonia), psychogenic dysphonia, malingering, and other conditions.

Fatigue of the voice is inability to continue to speak or sing for extended periods without change in vocal quality and/or control. The voice may show fatigue by becoming hoarse, losing range, changing timbre, breaking into different registers, or exhibiting other uncontrolled aberrations. A well-trained singer should be able to sing for several hours without vocal fatigue. Voice fatigue may occur through more than one mechanism.

Volume disturbance may manifest as inability to sing loudly or inability to sing softly. Most volume problems are secondary to intrinsic limitations of the voice or technical errors in voice use, although hormonal changes, aging, and neurologic disease are other causes. Superior laryngeal nerve paralysis impairs the ability to speak or sing loudly. This is a frequently unrecognized consequence of herpes infection (cold sores) and Lyme disease and may be precipitated by any viral upper respiratory tract infection.

Prolonged warm-up time, especially in the morning, is most often caused by reflux laryngitis, also called laryngopharyngeal reflux (LPR). Tickling or choking during singing is most often a symptom of an abnormality of the vocal fold's leading edge. The symptom of tickling or choking should contraindicate singing or other vigorous voice use until the vocal folds have been examined. Pain while singing can indicate vocal fold lesions, laryngeal joint arthritis, infection, or gastric acid reflux irritation of the arytenoid region. However, pain is caused much more commonly by voice abuse or misuse with excessive muscular activity in the neck rather than an acute abnormality on the leading edge of a vocal fold. In the absence of other symptoms, these patients do not generally require immediate cessation of phonation pending medical examination. However, sudden onset of pain (usually sharp pain) while singing or speaking may be associated with a mucosal tear or a vocal fold hemorrhage and warrants voice conservation pending laryngeal examination.

Do You Have Any Pressing Voice Commitments?

If a singer or professional speaker (eg, actor, politician) seeks treatment at the end of a busy performance season and has no pressing engagements, management of the voice problem should be relatively conservative and designed to ensure long-term protection of the larynx, the most delicate part of the voice mechanism. However, the physician and patient rarely have this luxury. Most often, the voice professional needs treatment within a week of an important engagement and sometimes within less than a day.

Tell Me About Your Voice Career, Long-Term Goals, and the Importance of Your Voice Quality and Upcoming Commitments

To choose a treatment program, the physician must understand the importance of the patient's voice and his or her long-term career plans, the importance of the upcoming voice commitment, and the consequences of canceling the engagement. Injudicious prescription of voice rest can be almost as damaging to a voice career as injudicious performance.

How Much Voice Training Have You Had?

Establishing how long a singer, actor or other speaker has been performing seriously is important, especially if his or her active performance career predates the beginning of voice training. Active untrained singers, actors and other professional speakers frequently develop undesirable techniques that are difficult to modify. Extensive voice use without training or premature training with inappropriate repertoire may underlie persistent vocal difficulties later in life.

Under What Kinds of Conditions Do You Use Your Voice?

The Lombard effect is the tendency to increase voice intensity in response to increased background noise. A well-trained singer learns to compensate for this tendency and to avoid singing at unsafe volumes. Singers of classical music usually have such training and frequently perform with only a piano, a situation in which the balance can be controlled well. However, singers performing in large halls, with orchestras, or in operas early in their careers tend to oversing and strain their voices. Similar problems occur during outdoor concerts because of the lack of auditory feedback. This phenomenon is seen even more among "pop" singers.

Amateur singers are often no less serious about their music than are professionals, but generally they have less ability to compensate technically for illness or other physical impairment. Rarely does an amateur suffer a great loss from postponing a performance or permitting someone to sing in his or her place. In most cases, the amateur singer's best interest is served through conservative management directed at long-term maintenance of good vocal health.

How Much Do You Practice and Exercise Your Voice? How, When, and Where Do You Use Your Voice?

Vocal exercise is as essential to the vocalist as exercise and conditioning of other muscle systems are to other athletes. Proper voice practice incorporates scales and specific exercises designed to maintain and develop the vocal apparatus. Simply acting or singing songs or giving performances without routine studious concentration on voice technique is not adequate for the vocal performer.

The physician should be aware of common habits and environments that are often associated with abusive voice behavior and should ask about them routinely. Screaming at sports events and at children is among the most common. Extensive voice use in noisy environments also tends to be abusive. Such environments include noisy rooms, cars, airplanes, sports facilities, and other locations where background noise or acoustic design impairs auditory feedback. Dry, dusty surroundings may alter vocal fold secretions through dehydration or contact irritation, altering voice function.

Are You Aware of Misusing or Abusing Your Voice During Singing?

A detailed discussion of voice technique in singing is beyond the scope of this chapter. The most common technical errors involve excessive muscle tension in the tongue, neck, and larynx; inadequate abdominal support; and excessive volume. Inadequate preparation can be a devastating source of voice abuse and may result from limited practice, limited rehearsal of a difficult piece, or limited vocal training for a given role.

Are You Aware of Misusing or Abusing Your Voice During Speaking?

Voice abuse and/or vocal misuse should be suspected particularly in patients who complain of voice fatigue associated with voice use, whose voices are worse at the end of a working day or week, and in any patient who is chronically hoarse. Technical errors in voice use may be the primary etiology of a voice complaint, or it may have developed secondarily due to a patient's effort to compensate for voice disturbance from another cause.

Do You Have Pain When You Talk or Sing?

Odynophonia, or pain caused by phonation, can be disturbing. It is not uncommon, but relatively little has been written on this subject. Laryngologists should be familiar with the diagnosis and treatment of at least a few of the most common causes.

What Kind of Physical Condition Are You In?

Phonation is an athletic activity that requires good conditioning and coordinated interaction of numerous physical functions. Maladies of any part of the body may be reflected in the voice. Failure to maintain good abdominal muscle tone and respiratory endurance through exercise is particularly harmful because deficiencies in those areas undermine the power source of the voice. Patients generally attempt to compensate for such weaknesses by using inappropriate muscle groups, particularly in the neck, causing voice dysfunction.

How Is Your Hearing?

Hearing loss can cause substantial problems for singers and other professional voice users. This may be true especially when the voice patient is unaware that he or she has hearing loss. Consequently, not only should voice patients be asked about hearing loss, tinnitus, vertigo, and family history of hearing loss, but it is also helpful to inquire of spouses, partners, friends, or others who may have accompanied the patient to the office whether they have suspected a hearing impairment in the patient. Obtaining an audiogram may be appropriate in any voice patient [6].

Have You Noted Voice or Bodily Weakness, Tremor, Fatigue, or Loss of Control?

Even minor neurologic disorders may be extremely disruptive to voice function. Specific questions should be asked to rule out neuromuscular and neurologic diseases such as myasthenia gravis, Parkinson disease, tremors, other movement disorders, spasmodic dysphonia, multiple sclerosis, central nervous system neoplasm, and other serious maladies that may be present with voice complaints.

Do You Have Allergy or Cold Symptoms?

Acute upper respiratory tract infection causes inflammation of the mucosa, alters mucosal secretions, and makes the mucosa more vulnerable to injury. Coughing and throat clearing are particularly traumatic vocal activities and may worsen or provoke hoarseness associated with a cold. Postnasal drip and allergy may produce the same response.

Do You Have Breathing Problems, Especially After Exercise?

Respiratory problems are especially important in voice patients. Even mild respiratory dysfunction may adversely affect the power source of the voice [7]. Occult asthma may be particularly troublesome [8]. A complete respiratory history should be obtained in most patients with voice complaints, and pulmonary function testing is often advisable.

Have You Been Exposed to Environmental Irritants?

Any mucosal irritant can disrupt the delicate voice mechanism. Allergies to dust and mold are aggravated commonly during rehearsals and performances in concert halls, especially older theaters and concert halls, because of numerous curtains, backstage trappings, and dressing room facilities that are rarely cleaned thoroughly. Nasal obstruction and erythematous conjunctivae suggest generalized mucosal irritation. The drying effects of cold air and dry heat also may affect mucosal secretions, leading to decreased lubrication, a "scratchy" voice, and tickling cough.

A history of recent travel suggests other sources of mucosal irritation. The air in airplanes is extremely dry, and airplanes are noisy [9]. Environmental changes also can be disruptive. Las Vegas is infamous for the mucosal irritation caused by its dry atmosphere and smoke-filled rooms. In fact, the resultant complex of hoarseness, vocal "tickle," and fatigue is referred to as "Las Vegas voice." A history of recent travel also should suggest jet lag and generalized fatigue, which may be potent detriments to good vocal function.

Environmental pollution is responsible for the presence of toxic substances and conditions encountered daily. Inhalation of toxic pollutants may affect the voice adversely by direct laryngeal injury, by causing pulmonary dysfunction that results in voice maladies, or through impairments elsewhere in the vocal tract. Ingested substances, especially those that have neurolaryngologic effects, may also affect the voice adversely. Nonchemical environmental pollutants such as noise can cause voice abnormalities, as well.

Do You Smoke, Live with a Smoker, or Work Around Smoke?

The effects of smoking on voice performance were reviewed by Anticaglia et al. Smoking tobacco is the number one cause of preventable death in the United States, as well as the leading cause of heart disease, stroke, emphysema, and cancer. The Centers for Disease Control and Prevention (CDC) attributes approximately 442,000 premature (shortened life expectancy) deaths annually in the United States to smoking, which is more than the combined incidence of deaths caused by highway accidents, fires, murders, illegal drugs, suicides, and AIDS [10]. Approximately four million deaths per year worldwide result from smoking, and if this trend continues, by 2030, this figure will increase to about 10 million deaths globally [11]. In addition to causing life-threatening diseases, smoking impairs a great many body systems, including the vocal tract. Harmful consequences of smoking or being exposed to smoke influence voice performance adversely.

Tobacco smoke can damage the lungs' parenchyma and the exchange of air through respiration. Cigarette manufacturers add hundreds of ingredients to their tobacco products to improve taste, to make smoking seem milder and easier to inhale, and to prolong burning and shelf life [12]. More than 3000 chemical compounds have been identified in tobacco smoke, and more than 60 of these compounds are carcinogens [13]. Most smokers want to stop, yet only a small percentage are successful in quitting cigarettes; the majority who quit relapse into smoking once again [14]. Tar and carbon monoxide are among the disease-causing components in tobacco products. The tar in cigarettes exposes the individual to a greater risk of bronchitis, emphysema, and lung cancer. These chemicals affect the entire vocal tract as well as the cardiovascular system.

An important component of voice quality is the symmetrical, unencumbered vibration of the true vocal folds. Anything that prevents the epithelium covering the vocal folds from vibrating or affects the loose connective tissue under the epithelium (in the superficial layer of the lamina propria known as the Reinke's space) can cause dysphonia. Cigarette smoking can cause the epithelium of the true vocal folds to become red and swollen, develop whitish discolorations (leukoplakia) sometimes with vocal fold stiffness, undergo chronic inflammatory changes, or develop squamous metaplasia or dysplasia (tissue changes from normal to a potentially malignant state). In chronic smokers, the voice may become husky due to the accumulation of fluid in Reinke's space (Reinke's edema). These alterations in structure can interfere with voice production by changing the biomechanics of the vocal folds and their vibratory characteristics. In severe cases, cancer can deform and immobilize the vocal folds.

Cigarette smoking also causes cancer of the nasopharynx [15] which can alter the vocal tract, as well as abnormalities of the tongue and lips that can impair articulation [16]. Smokeless "spit" tobacco is highly addictive, and users who dip 8 to 10 times a day may get the same nicotine exposure as those who smoke 1½ to 2 packs of cigarettes per day [17]. Smokeless tobacco has been associated with gingivitis, cheek carcinoma, and cancer of the larynx and hypopharynx.

Exposure to environmental tobacco smoke (ETS), also called secondhand smoke, sidestream smoke, or passive smoke, accounts for an estimated 3000 lung cancer deaths and approximately 35,000 deaths in the United States from heart disease in nonsmoking adults [18].

Secondhand smoke is the "passive" inhalation of tobacco smoke from environmental sources such as smoke given off by pipes, cigars, cigarettes (side-stream), or the smoke exhaled from the lungs of smokers and inhaled by other people (mainstream). Passive smoke contains a mixture of thousands of chemicals, some of which are known to cause cancer. The National Institutes of Health (NIH) lists ETS as a "known" carcinogen, and the more one is exposed to secondhand smoke, the greater the risk [19]. People who are exposed routinely to secondhand smoke are at risk for lung cancer, heart disease, respiratory infection, and an increased number of asthma attacks [20].

Do Any Foods Seem to Affect Your Voice?

Traditionally, singers avoid milk and ice cream before performances. In many people, these foods seem to increase the amount and viscosity of mucosal secretions. Allergy and casein have been implicated, but no satisfactory explanation has been established. Chocolate may have the same effect and should be viewed similarly. Chocolate also contains caffeine, which may aggravate reflux or cause tremor. Highly spiced foods also may cause mucosal irritation. In addition, they seem to aggravate reflux laryngitis. Coffee and other beverages containing caffeine also aggravate reflux and may promote dehydration and/or alter secretions and necessitate frequent throat clearing in some people. Fad diets, especially rapid weight-reducing diets, are notorious for causing voice problems.

Do You Have Morning Hoarseness, Bad Breath, Excessive Phlegm, a Lump in Your Throat, or Heartburn?

Laryngopharyngeal reflux is especially common among singers and trained speakers because of the high intraabdominal pressure associated with proper support and because of lifestyle. Singers frequently perform at night. Many vocalists refrain from eating before performances because a full stomach can compromise effective abdominal support. They typically compensate by eating heartily at postperformance gatherings late at night and then go to bed with a full stomach. Chronic irritation of arytenoid and vocal fold mucosa by reflux of gastric secretions may occasionally be associated with dyspepsia or pyrosis. However, the key features of this malady are bitter taste and halitosis on awakening in the morning, a dry or "coated" mouth, often a scratchy sore throat or a feeling of a "lump in the throat," hoarseness, and the need for prolonged vocal warm-up.

Do You Have Trouble with Your Bowels or Belly?

Any condition that alters abdominal function, such as muscle spasm, constipation or diarrhea, interferes with support and may result in a voice complaint. These symptoms may accompany infection, anxiety, various gastroenterological diseases, Fibromyalgia and other maladies.

Are You Under Particular Stress or in Therapy?

The human voice is an exquisitely sensitive messenger of emotion. Highly trained voice professionals learn to control the effects of anxiety and other emotional stress on their voices under ordinary circumstances. However, in some instances, this training may break down, or a performer may be inadequately prepared to control the voice under specific stressful conditions. Preperformance anxiety is the most common example, but insecurity, depression, and other emotional disturbances also generally are reflected in the voice. Recent publications have highlighted the complexity and importance of psychological factors associated with voice disorders [21].

Do You Have Problems Controlling Your Weight? Are You Excessively Tired? Are You Cold When Other People Are Warm?

The human voice is extremely sensitive to endocrinologic changes. Many of these are reflected in alterations of fluid content in the lamina propria just beneath the laryngeal mucosa. This causes alterations in the bulk and shape of the vocal folds and results in voice change. Hypothyroidism [22–26] is a well-recognized cause of such voice disorders, although the mechanism is not understood fully. Hoarseness, vocal fatigue, muffling of the voice, loss of range, and a sensation of a lump in the throat may be present even with mild hypothyroidism. Thyrotoxicosis may result in similar voice disturbances [23]

Do You Have Menstrual Irregularity, Cyclical Voice Changes Associated with Menses, Recent Menopause, or Other Hormonal Changes or Problems?

Voice changes associated with sex hormones are encountered commonly in clinical practice and have been investigated more thoroughly than have other hormonal changes [27, 28]. Although a correlation appears to exist between sex hormone levels and depth of male voices (higher testosterone and lower estradiol levels in basses than in tenors) [27], the most important hormonal considerations in males occur during or related to puberty [29, 30]. Voice problems related to sex hormones are more common in female singers and have been studied for many years [31–47].

Do You Have Jaw Joint or Other Dental Problems?

Dental disease, especially temporomandibular joint (TMJ) dysfunction, introduces muscle tension in the head and neck, which is transmitted to the larynx directly through the muscular attachments between the mandible and the hyoid bone and indirectly as generalized increased muscle tension. These problems often result in decreased range, vocal fatigue, and change in the quality or placement of a voice

Do You or Your Blood Relatives Have Hearing Loss?

Hearing loss often is overlooked as a source of vocal problems. Auditory feedback is fundamental to speaking and singing. Interference with this control mechanism may result in altered vocal production, particularly if the person is unaware of the hearing loss. Distortion, particularly pitch distortion (diplacusis), may also pose serious problems for the singer. This appears to be due not only to aesthetic difficulties in matching pitch but also to voice strain that accompanies pitch shifts [48].

In addition to determining whether the patient has hearing loss, inquiry should also be made about hearing impairment occurring in family members, roommates, and other close associates. Speaking loudly to people who are hard of hearing can cause substantial, chronic voice strain.

Have You Suffered Whiplash or Other Bodily Injury?

Various bodily injuries outside the confines of the vocal tract may have profound effects on the voice. Whiplash, for example, commonly causes changes in technique, with consequent voice fatigue, loss of range, difficulty singing softly, and other problems. These problems derive from the neck muscle spasm, abnormal neck posturing secondary to pain, and consequent hyperfunctional voice use. Lumbar, abdominal, head, chest, supraglottic, and extremity injuries also may affect voice technique and be responsible for the dysphonia that prompted the voice patient to seek medical attention.

Did You Undergo Any Surgery Prior to the Onset of Your Voice Problems?

A history of laryngeal surgery in a voice patient is a matter of great concern. It is important to establish why the surgery was done, by whom it was done, whether intubation was necessary, and whether voice therapy was instituted pre-or postoperatively if the surgery was for a voice disorder. If the vocal dysfunction that sent the patient to the physician's office dates from the immediate postoperative period, surgical trauma must be suspected.

What Medications and Other Substances Do You Use?

A history of alcohol abuse suggests the probability of poor voice technique. Intoxication results in incoordination and decreased awareness, which undermine vocal discipline designed to optimize and protect the voice.

Patients frequently acquire antihistamines to help control "postnasal drip" or other symptoms. The drying effect of antihistamines may result in decreased vocal fold lubrication, increased throat clearing, and irritability leading to frequent coughing. Antihistamines may be helpful to some voice patients, but they must be used with caution.

When a voice patient seeking the attention of a physician is already taking antibiotics, it is important to find out the dose and the prescribing physician, if any, as well as whether the patient frequently treats himself or herself with inadequate courses of antibiotics often supplied by colleagues.

Diuretics are also popular among some performers. They often are prescribed by gynecologists at the vocalist's request to help deplete excess water in the premenstrual period. They are not effective in this for this purpose, because they cannot diurese the protein-bound water in the laryngeal ground substance.

Hormone use, especially use of oral contraceptives, must be mentioned specifically during the physician's inquiry. Women frequently do not mention them routinely when asked whether they are taking any medication. Vitamins are also frequently not mentioned. Most vitamin therapy seems to have little effect on the voice. However, high-dose vitamin C (5 to 6 g/day), which some people use to prevent upper respiratory tract infections, seems to act as a mild diuretic and may lead to dehydration and xerophonia [49].

Cocaine use is common, especially among pop musicians. This drug can be extremely irritating to the nasal mucosa, causes marked vasoconstriction, and may alter the sensorium, resulting in decreased voice control and a tendency toward voice abuse.

Many pain medications (including aspirin and ibuprofen), psychotropic medications, and others may be responsible for a voice complaint. So far, no adverse voice effects have been reported with selective COX-2 inhibiting anti-inflammatory medications (which do not promote bleeding, as do other nonsteroidal anti-inflammatory medicines and aspirin) such as celecoxib (Celebrex; Pfizer, Inc., New York, New York) and valecoxib (Bextra; Pharmacia Corp, New York, New York). However this group of drugs has other side effects, and should be taken only under the care of a physician [50]. The voice effects of other new medications such as sildenafil citrate (Viagra; Pfizer, Inc) and related medicines, as well as medications used to induce abortion remain understudied and largely unknown, plausible that such medication may affect voice function, at least temporarily. Laryngologists should be familiar with the laryngologic effects of the many substances ingested medically and recreationally.

Physical Examination

Physical examination must include a thorough ear, nose, and throat evaluation and assessment of general physical condition. A patient who is extremely obese or appears fatigued, agitated, emotionally stressed, or otherwise generally ill, for example, has increased potential for voice dysfunction.

This could be due to altered abdominal support, loss of fine motor control of laryngeal muscles, decreased bulk of the submucosal vocal fold ground substance, change in the character of mucosal secretions, or other similar mechanisms. Any physical condition that impairs the normal function of the abdominal musculature should be suspect as cause for dysphonia. Some conditions, such as pregnancy, are obvious; however, a sprained ankle or broken leg that requires the singer to balance in an unaccustomed posture may distract him or her from maintaining good abdominal support and thereby result in voice dysfunction.

Complete Ear, Nose, and Throat Examination

Examination of the ears must include assessment of hearing acuity. Even a relatively slight hearing loss may result in voice strain as a singer or speaker tries to balance his or her vocal intensity with that of associate performers. The effect is most pronounced with sensorineural hearing loss. Diplacusis, distortion of pitch perception, makes voice strain even worse. Hearing loss in a spouse may be problematic, as well, if the voice professional strains vocally to communicate.

During an ear, nose, and throat examination, the conjunctivae and sclerae should be observed routinely for erythema that suggests allergy or irritation, for pallor that suggests anemia, and for other abnormalities such as jaundice. These observations may reveal the problem reflected in the vocal tract even before the larynx is visualized.

The nose should be assessed for patency of the nasal airway, character of the nasal mucosa, and nature of secretions, if any. Examination of the oral cavity should include careful attention to the tonsils and lymphoid tissue in the posterior pharyngeal wall, as well as to the mucosa. Diffuse lymphoid hypertrophy associated with a complaint of "scratchy" voice and irritative cough may indicate infection. The amount and viscosity of mucosal and salivary secretions also should be noted. Xerostomia is particularly important.

Dental examination should focus not only on oral hygiene but also on the presence of wear facets suggestive of bruxism. Bruxism is a clue to excessive tension and may be associated with dysfunction of the temporomandibular joints, which should also be assessed routinely. Thinning of the enamel of the central incisors in a normal or underweight patient may be a clue to bulimia. However, it also may also result from excessive ingestion of lemons, which some singers eat to help thin their secretions.

The neck should be examined for masses, restriction of movement, excess muscle tension and/or spasm, and scars from prior neck surgery or trauma. Laryngeal vertical mobility is also important. Particular attention should be paid to the thyroid gland. Examination of posterior neck muscles and range of motion should not be neglected. The cranial nerves should be examined routinely.

Laryngeal Examination

The range, ease, volume, and quality of the speaking voice should be noted. If the examination is not being conducted in the patient's native language, the physician should be sure to listen to a sample of the patient's mother tongue, as well. Voice use is often different under the strain or habits of foreign language use. Rating scales of the speaking voice may be helpful. The classification proposed by the Japanese Society of Logopedics and Phoniatrics (GRBAS) is one of the most widely used [51] as is the CAPE-V [52]. Physicians should at least be able to discriminate substantial differences in range and timbre, such as between bass and tenor, or alto and soprano. Although the correlation between speaking and singing voices is not perfect, a speaker with a low, comfortable bass voice who reports that he is a tenor may be misclassified and singing inappropriate repertoire with consequent voice strain. This judgment should be deferred to an expert, but the observation should lead the physician to make the appropriate referral. Excessive volume or obvious strain during speaking clearly indicates that voice abuse is present and may be contributing to the patient's voice complaint. The speaking voice can be evaluated more consistently and accurately using standardized reading passages, and such assessments are performed routinely by speech-language pathologists, phoniatricians, singing voice specialists and sometimes by laryngologists.

Any patient with a voice complaint should be examined by indirect laryngoscopy at least. It is not possible to judge voice range, quality, or other voice attributes by inspection of the vocal folds. However, the presence or absence of mass lesions, contact ulcers, hemorrhage, erythema, paresis or paralysis, arytenoid erythema (often reflux), and other anatomic abnormalities must be established. The mirror or a laryngeal telescope often provides a better view of the posterior portion of the endolarynx than is obtained with flexible endoscopy. Stroboscopic examination adds substantially to diagnostic abilities.

A laryngeal telescope may be combined with a stroboscope to provide excellent visualization of the vocal folds and related structures. The combination of a telescope and stroboscope provides optimal magnification and optical quality for assessment of vocal fold vibration. However, it is generally performed with the tongue in a fixed position, and the nature of the examination does not permit assessment of the larynx during normal phonatory gestures. Flexible laryngoscopy allows inspection of the vocal folds in patients whose vocal folds are difficult to visualize indirectly. In addition, it permits observation of the voice mechanism in a more natural posture than does indirect laryngoscopy, permitting sophisticated dynamic voice assessment. In the hands of an experienced endoscopist, this method may provide a great deal of information about both speaking and singing techniques.

Rigid endoscopy under general anesthesia may be reserved for the rare patient whose vocal folds cannot be assessed adequately by other means or for patients who need surgical procedures to remove or biopsy laryngeal lesions.

Objective Tests

Reliable, valid, objective analysis of the voice is extremely important and is an essential part of a comprehensive physical examination [1]. It is as valuable to the laryngologist as audiometry is to the otologist [1]. Familiarity with some of the measures and technological advances currently available is helpful. This information is covered in greater detail elsewhere [1].

Strobovideolaryngoscopy and Other Techniques to Evaluate Vocal Fold Vibration

Under continuous light, the vocal folds vibrate approximately 250 times/s while phonating at middle C. The human eye cannot discern the necessary details during such rapid motion. The vibratory margin may be assessed through high-speed photography, strobovideolaryngoscopy, high-speed video, videokymography, electroglottography (EEG), or photoglottography. Strobovideolaryngoscopy provides the necessary clinical information in a practical fashion, allowing routine slow-motion evaluation of the mucosal cover layer of the leading edge of the vocal fold. Stroboscopy does not provide a true slow-motion image, as obtained through high-speed photography, and stroboscopy works best for voices that are not severely dysphonic.

Measures of Phonatory Ability

Objective measures of phonatory ability are easy to use, readily available to the laryngologist, helpful in the evaluation of voice disorders, and quite useful in assessing the results of surgical treatment. Maximum phonation time is measured with a stopwatch. Frequency range of phonation is recorded in semitones and documents the voice range from the lowest note in the modal register (excluding vocal fry) to the highest falsetto note. This is the physiologic frequency range of phonation and disregards quality. The musical frequency range of phonation measures lowest to highest notes of musically acceptable quality. Tests for maximum phonation time, frequency ranges, and many of the other parameters also are useful.

Frequency limits of vocal register also may be measured. The registers are (from low to high) vocal fry, chest, mid, head, and falsetto. However, classification of registers is controversial, and many other classifications are used. Although the classification listed above is common among musicians, at present, most voice scientists prefer to classify registers as pulse, modal, and loft. Overlap of frequency among registers occurs routinely.

Testing the speaking fundamental frequency often reveals excessively low pitch, an abnormality associated with chronic voice abuse and development of vocal nodules. This parameter may be followed objectively throughout a course of voice therapy. Intensity range of phonation (IRP) has proven a less useful measure than frequency range.

Aerodynamic Measures

Traditional pulmonary function testing provides the most readily accessible measure of respiratory function. For singers and professional speakers with an abnormality caused by voice abuse/misuse, abnormal pulmonary function tests may confirm deficiencies in aerobic conditioning or reveal previously unrecognized asthma or other respiratory disorder [51]. Flow glottography with computer inverse filtering is also a practical and valuable diagnostic tool for assessing flow at the vocal fold level, evaluating the voice source, and imaging the balance between adductory forces and subglottal pressure [53]. It also has therapeutic value as a biofeedback tool.

Air volume is measured by the use of a mask fitted tightly over the face or by phonating into a mouthpiece while wearing a nose clamp. Measurements may be made using a spirometer, pneumotachograph, hot-wire anemometer or other technology. Glottal resistance cannot be measured directly, but it may be calculated from the mean flow rate and mean subglottal pressure.

Acoustic Analysis

Acoustic analysis equipment can determine frequency, intensity, harmonic spectrum, cycle-to-cycle perturbations in frequency (jitter), cycle-to-cycle perturbations in amplitude (shimmer), harmonics-to-noise ratios, breathiness index, and many other parameters. These data are useful for diagnosis and for outcomes assessment.

Laryngeal Electromyography

Electromyography (EMG) requires an electrode system, an amplifier, an oscilloscope, a loudspeaker, and a recording system [54]. Electrodes are placed transcutaneously into laryngeal muscles. EMG can be extremely valuable in confirming cases of vocal fold paresis, in differentiating paralysis from arytenoid dislocation, distinguishing recurrent laryngeal nerve paralysis from combined recurrent and superior nerve paralysis, diagnosing other more subtle neurolaryngologic pathology, detecting focal laryngeal myasthenia gravis, and documenting functional voice disorders and malingering. It is also recommended for needle localization when using botulinum toxin for treatment of spasmodic dysphonia and other conditions.

Psychoacoustic Evaluation

Because the human ear and brain are the most sensitive and complex analyzers of sound currently available, many researchers have tried to standardize and quantify psychoacoustic evaluation [3, 51, 52]. Unfortunately, even definitions of basic terms such as hoarseness and breathiness are still controversial. Psychoacoustic evaluation protocols and interpretations are not fully standardized. Consequently, although subjective psychoacoustic analysis of voice is of great value to the individual skilled clinician, it remains generally unsatisfactory for comparing research among laboratories or for reporting clinical results. It is useful clinically especially when performed by the same clinician repeatedly over time.

Assessment of Impact of a Voice Disorder

Measuring the impact of a voice disorder has always been challenging. However, recent advances have begun to address this problem. Validated instruments such as the Voice Handicap Index (VHI) [55] and modifications thereof are currently in clinical use and are likely to be used widely in future years.

Voice Impairment and Disability

Quantifying voice impairment and assigning a disability rating (percentage of whole person) remain controversial. This subject is still not addressed comprehensively even in the most recent editions of the American Medical Association's Guidelines for the Evaluation of Impairment and Disability (The Guides). The Guides still do not take into account the person's profession when calculating disability. Alternative approaches have been proposed [56], and advances in this complex arena are anticipated over the next few years.

Evaluation of the Singing Voice

The physician must be careful not to exceed the limits of his or her expertise, especially in caring for singers. However, if voice abuse or technical error is suspected, or if a difficult judgment must be reached on whether to allow a sick singer to perform, a brief observation of the patient's singing may provide invaluable information. Information on analysis of specific behaviors is available elsewhere.

Additional Examinations

A general physical examination should be performed whenever the patient's systemic health is questionable. Debilitating conditions such as mononucleosis may be noticed first by the singer as voice fatigue. A neurologic assessment may be particularly revealing. The physician must be careful not to overlook dysarthrias and dysphonias that are characteristic of movement disorders and of serious neurologic disease.

Following history and physical examination, physicians may suspect many etiologies for the voice complaint, some of which are discussed in Chap. 5. Depending upon the differential diagnosis, blood tests, imaging studies such as CT, MRI and fMRI, and other investigations may be appropriate. Blood studies may include complete blood count, fasting glucose, cholesterol, triglycerides, FTA-abs, Lyme titer, T3, T4, TSH, anti-thyroid peroxidase anybody, antithyroglobulin anybody, ANA, rheumatoid factor, sedimentation rate, anti-acetylcholine receptor anybody, anti-striatal muscle antibody, MuSK antibody, other tests for autoimmune diseases, B12, folate and others such as tests specific to Fibromyalgia discussed later in in this book. The importance of comprehensive laboratory evaluation has been established in the literature for vocal fold paresis and paralysis, and such assessment has been shown to reveal diagnoses that would have been missed without comprehensive assessment [57]. Thorough assessment is important not only for movement disorders, but also for all of the conditions that might bring a patient to medical attention for a voice complaint.

Acknowledgments Modified in part from Sataloff RT. Professional Voice: The Science and Art of Clinical Care, 4th Edition. San Diego, CA: Plural Publishing; 2017, with permission.

References

1. Sataloff RT. Professional singers: the science and art of clinical care. 4th ed. San Diego: Plural Publishing; 2017. p. 157–234, 259–308, 361–584
2. Sataloff RT. The human voice. Sci Am. 1992;267:108–15.
3. Sundberg J. The science of the singing voice. DeKalb: Northern Illinois University Press; 1987.
4. Ackerman R, Pfan W. Gerontology studies on the susceptibility to voice disorders in professional speakers. Folia Phoniatr (Basel). 1974;26:95–9.
5. von Leden H. Speech and hearing problems in the geriatric patient. J Am Geriatr Soc. 1977;25:422–6.
6. Hu A, Hofmann E, Davis J, Capo J, Sataloff RT. Hearing loss in singers: a preliminary study. J Voice. 2015;29(1):120–4.
7. Spiegel JR, Cohn JR, Sataloff RT, et al. Respiratory function in singers: medical assessment, diagnoses, treatments. J Voice. 1988;2:40–50.
8. Cohn JR, Sataloff RT, Spiegel JR, et al. Airway reactivity-induced asthma in singers (ARIAS). J Voice. 1991;5:332–7.
9. Feder RJ. The professional voice and airline flight. Otolaryngol Head Neck Surg. 1984;92:251–4.
10. Centers for Disease Control and Prevention. Annual smoking-attributable, mortality, years of potential life lost, and economic costs, United States—1995–1999. MMWR Morb Mortal Wkly Rep. 2005;54(25):625–8.
11. World Health Organization. World health report 1999. Geneva: World Health Organization; 1999.
12. United States Department of Health Services. Tobacco products fact sheet. Washington, DC: Government Printing Office; 2000.
13. National Cancer Institute. Environmental tobacco smoke. Fact sheet 3.9; 1999. https://cis.nci.nih.gov/fact/3_9.htm.
14. Centers for Disease Control and Prevention. Cigarette smoking among adults—United States, 1993. MMWR Morb Mortal Wkly Rep. 1994;3:925–9.
15. Chow WH, McLaughlin JK, Hrubec Z, et al. Tobacco use and nasopharyngeal carcinoma in a cohort of US veterans. Int J Cancer. 1993;55(4):538–40.
16. Casiglia J, Woo SB. A comprehensive view of oral cancer. Gen Dent. 2001;49(1):72–82.
17. Centers for Disease Control and Prevention. Determination of nicotine pH and moisture content of six U.S. commercial moist snuff products. MMWR Morb Mortal Wkly Rep. 1999;48(19):398.
18. American Cancer Society. Cancer facts and figures 2002. Atlanta: American Cancer Society; 2002.
19. National Toxicology Program. Report on carcinogens. 10th ed. Research Triangle Park: U.S. Department Health and Human Services, Public Health Service, National Toxicology Program; 2002. http://ehp.niehs.nih.gov/roc/toc10.html.

20. Academy of Pediatrics, Committee on Environmental Health. Environmental tobacco smoke; a hazard to children. Pediatrics. 1997;99(4):639–42.
21. Rosen DC, Sataloff JB, Sataloff RT. Psychology of voice disorders. 2nd ed. San Diego: Plural Publishing; 2021.
22. Gupta OP, Bhatia PL, Agarwal MK, et al. Nasal pharyngeal and laryngeal manifestations of hypothyroidism. Ear Nose Throat J. 1997;56:10–21.
23. Malinsky M, Chevrie-Muller, Cerceau N. Etude clinique et electrophysiologique des alterations de la voix au cours des thyrotoxioses. Ann Endocrinol (Paris). 1997;38:171–2.
24. Michelsson K, Sirvio P. Cry analysis in congenital hypothyroidism. Folia Phoniatr (Basel). 1976;28:40–7.
25. Ritter FN. The effect of hypothyroidism on the larynx of the rat. Ann Otol Rhinol Laryngol. 1964;67:404–16.
26. Ritter FN. Endocrinology. In: Paparella M, Shumrick D, editors. Otolaryngology, vol. I. Philadelphia: Saunders; 1973. p. 727–34.
27. Abitbol J, Abitbol P, Abitbol B. Sex hormones and the female voice. J Voice. 1999;13(3):424–46.
28. Zamponi V, Mazzilli R, Mazzilli F, Fantini M. Effect of sex hormones on human voice physiology: from childhood to senescence. Hormones (Athens). 2021;20(4):691–6.
29. Brodnitz F. The age of the castrato voice. J Speech Hear Disord. 1975;40:291–5.
30. Brodnitz F. Hormones and the human voice. Bull NY Acad Med. 1971;47:183–91.
31. Carroll C. Personal communication with Dr. Hans von Leden. Arizona State University at Tempe; 1992.
32. von Gelder L. Psychosomatic aspects of endocrine disorders of the voice. J Commun Disord. 1974;7:257–62.
33. Lacina O. Der Einfluss der menstruation auf die stimme der sangerinnen. Folia Phoniatr (Basel). 1968;20:13–24.
34. Wendler J. The influence of menstruation on the voice of the female singer. Folia Phoniatr (Basel). 1972;24:259–77.
35. Rodney J, Sataloff RT. The effects of hormonal contraception on the voice: history of its evolution in the literature. J Voice. 2016;30(6):726–30.
36. Dordain M. Etude Statistique de l'influence des contraceptifs hormonaux sur la voix. Folia Phoniatr (Basel). 1972;24:86–96.
37. Pahn J, Goretzlehner G. Voice changes following the use of oral contraceptives [in German]. Zentralbl Gynakol. 1978;100:341–6.
38. Schiff M. "The pill" in otolaryngology. Trans Am Acad Ophthalmol Otolaryngol. 1968;72:76–84.
39. von Deuster CV. Irreversible vocal changes in pregnancy [in German]. HNO. 1977;25:430–2.
40. Flach M, Schwickardi H, Simen R. Welchen einfluss haben menstruation and schwangerschaft auf die augsgebildete gesangsstimme? Folia Phoniatr (Basel). 1968;21:199–210.
41. Arndt HJ. Stimmstorungen nach Behandlung mit Androgenen und anabolen Hormonen. Munch Med Wochenschr. 1974;116:1715–20.
42. Bourdial J. Les troubles de la voix provoques par la therapeutique hormonale androgene. Ann Otolaryngol Chir Cervicofac. 1970;87:725–34.
43. Damste PH. Virilization of the voice due to anabolic steroids [in Dutch]. Ned Tijdschr Geneeskd. 1963;107:891–2.
44. Damste PH. Voice changes in adult women caused by virilizing agents. J Speech Hear Disord. 1967;32:126–32.
45. Saez S, Francoise S. Recepteurs d'androgenes: mise en evidence dans la fraction cytosolique de muqueuse normale et d'epitheliomas phryngolarynges humains. C R Acad Sci Hebd Seances Acad Sci D. 1975;280:935–8.
46. Vuorenkoski V, Lenko HL, Tjernlund P, et al. Fundamental voice frequency during normal and abnormal growth, and after androgen treatment. Arch Dis Child. 1978;53:201–9.
47. Imre V. Hormonell bedingte Stimmstorungen. Folia Phoniatr (Basel). 1968;20:394–404.

48. Sundberg J, Prame E, Iwarsson J. Replicability and accuracy of pitch patterns in professional singers. In: Davis PJ, Fletcher NH, editors. Vocal fold physiology: controlling chaos and complexity. San Diego: Singular Publishing Group; 1996. p. 291–306.
49. Lawrence VL. Medical care for professional voice (panel). In: Lawrence VL, editor. Transcripts from the annual symposium, care of the professional voice, vol. 3. New York: The Voice Foundation; 1978. p. 17–8.
50. Cannon CP. COX-2 inhibitors and cardiovascular risk. Science. 2012;336(6087):1386–7.
51. Hirano M. Clinical examination of the voice. New York: Springer; 1981.
52. Cohn JR, Sataloff RT, Spiegel JR, Fish JE, Kennedy K. Airway reactivity-induced asthma in singers (ARIAS). J Voice. 1991;5:332–7.
53. Kempster GB, Gerratt BR, Abbott KV, Barkmeier-Kramer J, Hillman R. Consensus auditory-perceptual evaluation of voice: development of a standardized clinical protocol. Ann J Speech Lang Pathol. 2009;18(2):124–32.
54. Sataloff RT, Mandel S, Heman-Ackah YD, Abaza M. Laryngeal electromyography. 3rd ed. San Diego: Plural Publishing; 2017.
55. Benninger MS, Syamal MN, Gardner GM, Jacobson BH. New dimensions in measuring voice treatment outcomes and quality of life. In: Sataloff RT, editor. Professional voice: the science and art of clinical care. 4th ed. San Diego: Plural Publishing; 2017. p. 547–58.
56. Sataloff RT. Voice impairment, disability, handicap, and medical-legal evaluation. In: Sataloff RT, editor. Professional voice: the science and art of clinical care. 4th ed. San Diego: Plural Publishing, Inc; 2017. p. 1741–54.
57. White M, Meenan K, Patel T, Jaworek A, Sataloff RT. Laboratory evaluation of vocal paralysis and paresis. J Voice. 2017;31(2):168–74.

Fibromyalgia: Clinical Presentation, Pathophysiology and Diagnosis

4

Abdul-latif Hamdan, Robert Thayer Sataloff, and Mary J. Hawkshaw

Clinical Presentation of Fibromyalgia and Associated Co-morbidities

Fibromyalgia (FM) is a medical condition characterized by diffuse pain with tender points at specific body sites. The pain is generalized and persistent for at least 3 months. Symptoms are precipitated by stress, increase in work load and external stimuli such as noise [1, 2]. The clinical presentation of Fibromyalgia is not limited to the musculoskeletal system but also may involve other systems in the body, as well. Commonly reported complaints aside from pain include body fatigue, dyspepsia, insomnia, sleep disturbance, decrease in cognitive capacity, imbalance, and mood alterations. Many of those complaints are attributed to coexistent morbidities that often are overlooked in patients diagnosed with FM. In a large cross-sectional study, *Vincent et al,* reported the presence of seven or more chronic medical conditions in more than 50% of patients with FM [3]. The most common comorbidities were chronic joint pain/degenerative arthritis and depression in 88.7% and 75.1% of the cases, respectively. The authors highlighted the need to account for those comorbidities in the treatment of patients with FM [3]. In a retrospective analysis of 411 FM patients engaged in a cognitive behavioral treatment program, *Rivera et al.* noted the presence of headache and obesity in 33.6% and 18.2% of the cases, respectively (The prevalence of obesity in Switzerland is 12%). Obesity and many other co-morbidities such as hypothyroidism and osteoarthritis were found to have adverse effects on treatment outcome [4]. *Lichtenstein et al.* reviewed the complexities of FM syndrome and noted the high prevalence of psychiatric and rheumatologic diseases in affected patients. The authors urged

A.-l. Hamdan et al., *Voice Disorders in Fibromyalgia*,
https://doi.org/10.1007/978-3-031-97751-0_4

consideration of these comorbidities in the management of FM [5]. *Acosta-Manzano et al.* conducted a cross-sectional study on 436 women with FM and found a higher risk for cardiovascular disease in comparison to controls. Predisposing factors included low level of cardiovascular fitness, increase in body fat and cigarette smoking [6]. *Su et al.* evaluated the risk of coronary heart disease (CHD) in 61.612 patients diagnosed with FM versus 184.834 reference subjects and noted a hazard ratio (HR) of 1.47 even after adjusting for age, gender, socio-economic status and other comorbidities such as anxiety and depression [7]. *Tseng et al.* investigated the link between FM and the risk of having a stroke in a large population-based cohort study. Stroke risk factors such as hypertension and hyperlipidemia were more prevalent in patients with FM versus controls, and the adjusted hazard ratio of having a stroke in FM taking into account these factors was 1.44, with a 95% CI. In patients less than 35 years old, the relative risk of stroke was 2.26-fold higher compared to controls. The findings of this study agreed with numerous reports in the literature asserting that neuropsychiatric diseases enhance the risk of developing a stroke particularly in the younger population [8].

The symptoms of Fibromyalgia are not always very distinctive. Pain may be localized or diffuse, and often is associated with other non-painful conditions. Physicians should be diligent about not overlooking comorbidities that may worsen the quality of life of affected patients and jeopardize treatment outcome.

Otolaryngological Manifestations of Fibromyalgia

Otolaryngologic manifestations of FM are common. Patients with FM may have ear, nose and throat symptoms that often are obscured by the complexity of the disease. The most common otolaryngologic symptoms are related to the ears. Otologic complaints include subjective hearing loss, tinnitus, hyperacusis and ear pain. Self-reported hearing impairment is prevalent in almost half patients with FM. The subjective decrease in hearing may or may not be substantiated by objective hearing loss on audiologic examination. *Bayzati et al.* investigated the prevalence of otologic symptoms in 24 female patients with FM and noted ear-related complaints in 47% of the cases. Tinnitus and hearing loss were reported in 16.7% and 12% of the cases, respectively. Vertigo was the most common symptom, although there was no significant difference in the auditory brain response (ABR) results between those with cochlea-vestibular symptoms and those without. It is worth noting that 23 out of the 24 patients had a normal audiogram [9]. *Koca et al.* investigated the otologic manifestations in 44 patients with FM and noted subjective tinnitus and subjective hearing loss in 63.6% and 45.4% of the cases, respectively. In contrast to the findings of Bayzati et al., audiometric evaluation showed elevated hearing threshold across all frequencies. Furthermore, the dizziness handicap score was higher in the FM group in comparison to controls [10]. Similarly, *Stranden et al.* reported that FM patients were 4.57 more likely to complain of subjective hearing loss in comparison to healthy subjects. The increased risk of hearing loss was not limited to FM patients but included also patients with other causes of diffuse musculoskeletal pain [11]. *Le et al.* found that FM increased the odds of having conductive and sensorineural hearing loss by 1.34 and 1.46-fold, respectively. Comorbidities such as diabetes, depression and hyperlipidemia increased the risk of hearing loss in affected subjects [12]. *Cil et al.* investigated tinnitus using the tinnitus handicap index in 101 patients with FM and found a prevalence of 74.3%. The authors reported improvement in tinnitus following the use of pregabalin or duloxetine, and highlighted the need for further investigation of the otologic complaints in patients with FM [13]. Another overlooked otologic symptom is hyperacusis. *Geisser et al.* demonstrated that patients with FM exhibited higher sensitivity to auditory stimuli than subjects with no FM. The study was conducted on 30 patients using both auditory and pressure stimuli [14].

Fibromyalgia also has been linked to rhinosinusitis. *Cleveland et al.* investigated 47 patients with allergic or non-allergic rhinitis and found that two out of five had widespread pain and at least 11 tender points diagnostic of FM. Although there was no correlation between the number of tender points and the positive skin tests to inhalant allergens, the authors highlighted the higher prevalence of FM in patients with nasal symptoms in comparison to the normal population [15]. *Gultuna et al.* examined 105 patients with allergic rhinitis and noted that 32.4% had FM based on the diagnostic criteria set by the American College of Rheumatology in 2010 [16]. Patients with allergic rhinitis and FM had worse scoring using the Nottingham Health Profile (NHP) in comparison to those without FM [17]. *Chester et al.* investigated 297 consecutive patients with chronic fatigue and body pain and noted a higher prevalence of rhinosinusitis in those with unexplained chronic fatigue in comparison to those with no body fatigue. The odds of having nasal obstruction, post-nasal drip and frontal headache were 4.3, 2.8 and 13.6, respectively [18].

Pharyngeal and laryngeal manifestation of FM are also common. That is not surprising given that the laryngopharyngeal complex is made of skeletal muscles similar to other musculoskeletal structures in the body affected by FM. FM patients suffer from a number of swallowing and voice symptoms [19, 20]. The basic physiologic functions of the larynx and related structures, namely phonation and swallowing, are affected by the disease itself and by the manifestation of many co-morbidities in patients with FM. A detailed review of the literature on the prevalence of voice and swallowing disorders is presented in Chap. 5 of this book.

Pathophysiology of Fibromyalgia

The pathophysiology of FM is complex and controversial. Many mechanisms have been suggested in the literature with no clear consensus. The most accepted explanation is central sensitization and alteration in pain processing [21]. The term "Central sensitization" has been introduced in the literature to explain the enhanced excitability witnessed in patients with FM. Three neurologic aberrances have been described; one is spontaneous in neural activity in the absence of a stimulus, second is the wide distribution of pain geographically in a given anatomic area, and third is temporal summation also referred to as "Wind-up" [22]. Neuroimaging studies using functional magnetic resonance imaging (MRI) showed increase in brain activity at rest in areas of the brain that were pain-relevant [23]. Other studies using the same imaging technique also showed higher cerebral blood flow following a painful peripheral stimulus in patients with FM in comparison to controls. Moreover, there were signs suggestive of dampening of the descending inhibitory pathways in FM patients [24]. These findings support the concept that pain in Fibromyalgia is also due to dysregulation in the descending efferent pain pathways responsible for modulation of response to pain [25, 26]. Central sensitization has been linked to the concept of "augmented" sensory stimuli in the central nervous system, which might explain hyperacusis in FM patients. The central mechanism of hyperacusis was highlighted in a review by *Suhnan et al.* which stressed the neural interactions between the nociceptive and auditory systems. The authors noted that the sensory convergence at the level of the thalamus in patients with central sensitivity could be responsible for hyperacusis [27]. In a study on hearing in FM patients, *Stranden et al.* noted that central sensitization was not limited to alteration in pain processing but to alteration in the perception of other internal and external stimuli, which might explain hyperacusis in some patients [11]. *Bayazit et al.* attributed the neurotologic symptoms to neural disintegration and abnormality in neural mediators leading to abnormal perception of external stimuli [9].

In attempt to understand better the complexity of FM and its varied clinical presentation, researchers explored a peripheral origin for pain in FM in addition to its well-known central component. Many histology studies have demonstrated the presence of small-fiber peripheral neuropathy (SFN) in affected patients. Based on a meta-analysis, it has been shown that almost 50% of FM patients have SFN [28, 29]. What supports the peripheral origin of pain in FM is the ability to transfer or reproduce the state of sensory hypersensibility in patients to animals. *Goebel et al.* were able to transfer FM symptoms from patient-derived IgG to mice [30]. Distinctive pathologic features of SFN in FM patients included neurogenic inflammatory changes and abnormalities in the Schwann cells [28].

There are many studies suggesting that FM, the peripheral phenotype at least, is incited by a state of chronic and diffuse inflammation. Inflammation and dysfunction in autoimmune response are thought to be the trigger in the underlying pathogenesis of FM. *Bazzichi et al.* examined the level of cytokines and other inflammatory markers in 80 patients diagnosed with FM and noted the presence of higher levels of IL-8, UL-10 and tumor necrosis factor-alpha (TNF-alpha) in comparison to controls. Moreover, there was a significant correlation between these inflammatory biomarkers and the clinical profile of the patients which supports the etiologic role of inflammation in the pathogenesis of FM [31]. *Bote et al.* investigated systemic inflammatory and neuroendocrine-stress biomarkers in 25 patients with FM and found high levels of CRP and IL-8 in all the subjects. There was also an increased level of inflammatory markers suggestive of dysregulation in the inflammatory and stress response in FM patients [32]. Similarly, *Kadetoff et al.* reported a high concentration of pro-inflammatory markers in the blood and CSF in FM. The elevated levels in response to pain were suggestive of activation of glia cells in affected patients [33].

There are also numerous studies highlighting impairment in the secretion of neuromodulators in Fibromyalgia patients. A reduction in the secretion of serotonin, a neurotransmitter that has inhibitory effect on pain pathways, has been reported by many. In one study, *Houvenagel et al.* demonstrated lower levels of serotonin in the cerebrospinal fluid of patients with Fibromyalgia in comparison to controls and patients with lower back pain [34]. These findings are in accord with many studies suggesting a disturbance in the hypothalamic-pituitary-adrenal axis associated with an increase in cortisol level and decrease in its diurnal fluctuation in patients with Fibromyalgia [33–56].

There is mounting evidence suggesting that FM is linked to muscle dysfunction. The question of whether FM is a muscular disease or not remains controversial. Alterations in muscle tissue structure and metabolism in affected patients have been demonstrated by many authors, with no consensus as to whether these are the cause or the result of this disorder. Numerous studies showed a decrease in the production of high-energy phosphate metabolites such as adenosine diphosphate (ADP) and adenosine triphosphate (ATP) in patients with FM, suggesting impairment in oxidative phosphorylation and alteration in protein expression [57, 58]. *E Lund et al.* investigated work capacity in FM patients and noted a reduction in inorganic phosphate and maximal oxygen uptake at maximal dynamic and static contractions. Those findings suggest that FM patients consume less energy rich phosphorous metabolites and reach anaerobic threshold faster than controls [59]. Those findings are in agreement with other investigators who showed high levels of anaerobic glycolysis end products in parallel with reduced oxidative metabolism. All these metabolic changes suggest the presence of alteration in the metabolic pathway and a delay in muscle recovery and repair [60]. Whether these changes are the cause of alteration in muscle morphology and function or the result of deconditioning is not known. Detraining, which is a common pattern in patients with Fibromyalgia also results in a decrease in high-energy phosphates which makes it hard to conclude whether these metabolic changes are the cause of the disease or the result of deconditioning that is observed commonly in diseased subjects.

There are many electrons microscopic studies documenting abnormalities in the shape and number of mitochondria [58]. Several studies have reported Coenzyme Q_{10} deficiency in blood mononuclear cells in Fibromyalgia. Coenzyme Q_{10} plays an essential role in the mitochondrial respiratory chain, a decrease in which had been shown to lead to oxidative stress [61]. *Beyaztas et al.* investigated the relation between oxidative stress and Fibromyalgia and found lower levels of total antioxidant status and higher levels of total oxidant status and oxidative stress index in Fibromyalgia patients in comparison to healthy controls. The authors concluded that reactive oxygen species have a negative effect on disease progression and treatment [62]. *Neval et al.* reported a significantly higher level of total oxidant status and a significantly lower level of plasma nitrate level and oxidant stress index in Fibromyalgia patients in comparison to controls. The authors stressed ~~on~~ the role of oxidative stress in the pathophysiology of Fibromyalgia [63].

Fibromyalgia is a neurologic disorder characterized by central sensitization and aberration in pain processing. Pain is amplified further by dysfunction in the descending inhibitory pathways responsible for downregulation of the pain signal. Muscle dysfunction, disorders in mitochondria function and oxidative stress also play a role in the pathophysiology of FM [64].

Diagnosis of Fibromyalgia

Accurate diagnosis of FM can be challenging given the multifaceted nature of this syndrome. The clinical assessment by the primary treating physician remain the most important determinant. Laboratory testing and imaging studies are warranted to exclude other systemic conditions that may mimic or co-exist with FM. Some of the most commonly ordered tests are complete blood count (CBC), renal and lever function tests, erythrocyte sedimentation rate and C-reactive protein. Other commonly performed tests include thyroid hormone tests to rule out hyperthyroidism and virologic serologic tests to exclude viral infectious agents linked to Fibromyalgia such as Ebstein-Barr virus (EBV), Cytomegalovirus (CMV) and Human Immunodeficiency virus (HIV) [65].

Several screening and diagnostic criteria for FM have been described in the literature over the last three to four decades. In 1990, the American College of Rheumatology (ACR) set the first criteria to diagnose FM, namely the presence of widespread pain for at least 3 months, in addition to point tenderness on digital palpation [66, 67]. The main limitation of these criteria was overlooking other symptoms and diseases of FM in addition to performing the tender point examination [68, 69]. To that end, in 2010 the ACR criteria were revised to include systemic complaints. Other domains such as emotional and physical functioning, as well as the overall well-being of the patient have been included in the assessment of suspected patients. The symptom severity scale (SSS) has been introduced to gauge the presence and severity of somatic symptoms, cognitive symptoms and other complaints like fatigue and waking unfreshened. The SSS was coupled with the Widespread Pain Index (WPI) using a Fibromyalgia score that ranges from 0–31, with a score above 13 being diagnostic of FM with a sensitivity and specificity of 91.8% and 96.6%, respectively [70–72]. A main limitation of this revision was not accounting for the spatial distribution of pain and the non-specificity of the widespread pain [73]. In 2016, the ACR criteria were revised again, and one of the requirements for diagnosis of FM was the presence of generalized pain in 4 to 5 distinct regions of the body. A WPI score above or equal to 7 and a SSS above or equal to 5 were one of the diagnostic criteria. Given the complexity of the disease, the coexistence of other diseases remained in the clinical diagnosis of this syndrome and were not excluded [16]. Other diagnostic criteria such as the Analgesic, Anesthetic, and Addiction Clinical Trial Translations Innovations Opportunities and Networks (ACTTION)-American Pain Society Pain Taxonomy (AAPT), and later the Fibromyalgia Assessment Status (FAS) criteria also were introduced, each with its advantages and limitations [74, 75].

Given the subjectivity and controversy in the diagnosis of FM which left a high percentage of patients underdiagnosed, numerous studies using more objective indicators have emerged [76]. These objective indicators included the presence of genetic and epigenetic markers. Genetic factors have been reported to be responsible for FM in almost half of patients. This was substantiated by the clustering of FM cases and the increased risk of FM among family members. Several genes have been identified among which are the SS genotype of the serotonin transporter (5-HTT) gene, the dopamine D4 receptor gene which has been shown to be reduced in affected patients [77], and the catechol-O-methyltransferase (COMT). High frequency of polymorphisms in metabolism genes have been also described [78].

The testing for molecular and non-molecular biologic markers has expanded to improve the screening and diagnosis of FM. *Crofford et al.* investigated the level of hormones related to the hypothalamic-pituitary-axis (HPA) in 12 patients with FM and found lower 24-h urine free cortisol and a significant decrease in the integrated cortisol response (net) to ovone corticotropin-releasing hormone suggestive of disturbance in the HPA axis function [79]. *Anderberg et al.* explored the link between neuropeptide Y (NPY) and FM symptoms and found higher levels in comparison to controls. The authors concluded that FM patients suffer from alteration the NPY activity in parallel with the perturbation in the HPA axis, which could be the result of repeated stress [80]. Along the same line, *Iannucelli et al.* evaluated the serum NPY level in patients with FM versus patients with tension headache and noted a significant difference between the two groups. There were higher levels of Interleukin (IL)-1RA, IL-6, IL-10 and tumor necrosis factor-alpha in comparison to patients with tension-type headache. The authors noted that the alteration in the cytokines and neurotransmitters may be partially responsible for the disturbance in pain modulation in affected patients [81]. *Valdes et al.* assessed the brain metabolite patterns in 28 patients with FM using magnetic resonance spectroscopy techniques. The results showed higher levels of glutamate/glutamine (Glx) compounds and Glx:creatinine ratio in comparison to controls. These findings suggested the presence of dysfunction in the processing of emotion in addition to the dysfunction in pain processing [82]. Another marker used for the diagnosis of FM is the brain derived neurotrophic factor (BDNF). *Sarchielli et al.* investigated the CSF level of nerve growth factor and BDNF in 20 patients with FM and noted higher levels in comparison to controls. Moreover, there was a positive correlation between CSF values of BDNF and glutamate which suggested new pathogenic mechanisms [83]. These results concur with those of *Laske et al.* who reported higher level of serum BDNF in FM patients in comparison to healthy controls [84].

The link between FM and anti-polymer antibody also has been explored by numerous authors highlighting the co-existence of many autoimmune diseases such as Sjogren syndrome, systemic lupus erythematosus and thyroid diseases such as Hashimoto thyroiditis [85, 86]. In another study exploring autoimmune and rheumatic disorders in FM patients, Klein et al. reported autoantibodies to serotonin, gangliosides and phospholipids in 70% of cases [87]. *Bazzichi et al.* examined the plasma level of 20 amino acids in 34 patients with FM and found lower level of seven in comparison to controls. The authors alluded to a possible defect in the absorption of many amino acids in FM patients [88]. Many hypothesized that the deficiency in amino acids could be responsible for the decrease in energy supply and disturbance in protein synthesis [88, 89].

In summary, FM is not a single disease but a spectrum that encompass disturbances in many systems in the body. The diagnosis relies on patients' self-reported complaints and clinical assessment. Serologic biomarkers can be screened to improve diagnosis in suspected patients. Future research is needed to elucidate the systemic presentation of FM.

References

1. Ablin J, Neumann L, Buskila D. Pathogenesis of fibromyalgia—a review. Joint Bone Spine. 2008;75(3):273–9.
2. Clauw D, Sarzi-Puttini P, Pellegrino G, Shoenfeld Y. Is fibromyalgia an autoimmune disorder? Autoimmun Rev. 2024;23(1):103424.
3. Vincent A, Whipple MO, McAllister SJ, et al. A cross-sectional assessment of the prevalence of multiple chronic conditions and medication use in a sample of community-dwelling adults with fibromyalgia in olmstead county minnesota. BMJ Open. 2015;5:e006681.
4. Rivera FA, Munipalli B, Allman ME, et al. A retrospective analysis of the prevalence and impact of associated comorbidities on fibromyalgia outcomes in a tertiary care center. Front Med (Lausanne). 2024;10:1301944.
5. Lichtenstein A, Tiosano S, Amital H. The complexities of fibromyalgia and its comorbidities. Curr Opin Rheumatol. 2018;30(1):94–100.
6. Acosta-Manzano P, Segura-Jiménez V, Estévez-López F, et al. Do women with fibromyalgia present higher cardiovascular disease risk profile than healthy women? The al-Ándalus project. Clin Exp Rheumatol. 2017;35(Suppl 105(3)):61–7.
7. Su CH, Chen JH, Lan JL, et al. Increased risk of coronary heart disease in patients with primary fibromyalgia and those with concomitant comorbidity-a Taiwanese population-based cohort study. PLoS One. 2015;10(9):e0137137.
8. Tseng CH, Chen JH, Wang YC, et al. Increased risk of stroke in patients with fibromyalgia: a population-based cohort study. Medicine (Baltimore). 2016;95(8):e2860.
9. Bayazit YA, Gürsoy S, Ozer E, et al. Neurotologic manifestations of the fibromyalgia syndrome. J Neurol Sci. 2002;196(1–2):77–80.
10. Koca TT, Seyithanoglu M, Sagiroglu S, et al. Frequency of audiological complaints in patients with fibromyalgia syndrome and its relationship with oxidative stress. Niger J Clin Pract. 2018;21(10):1271–7.
11. Stranden M, Solvin H, Fors EA, et al. Are persons with fibromyalgia or other musculoskeletal pain more likely to report hearing loss? A HUNT study. BMC Musculoskelet Disord. 2016;17(1):477.
12. Le TP, Tzeng YL, Muo CH, et al. Risk of hearing loss in patients with fibromyalgia: a nationwide population-based retrospective cohort study. PLoS One. 2020;15(9):e0238502.
13. Cil ÖÇ, Zateri C, Güçlü O, et al. The effect of fibromyalgia treatment on tinnitus. Am J Otolaryngol. 2020;41(3):102390.
14. Geisser ME, Glass JM, Rajcevska LD, et al. A psychophysical study of auditory and pressure sensitivity in patients with fibromyalgia and healthy controls. J Pain. 2008;9(5):417–22.
15. Cleveland CH Jr, Fisher RH, Brestel EP, et al. Chronic rhinitis: an underrecognized association with fibromyalgia. Allergy Proc. 1992;13(5):263–7.
16. Wolfe F, Clauw DJ, Fitzcharles MA, Goldenberg DL, Häuser W, Katz RL, et al. 2016 Revisions to the 2010/2011 fibromyalgia diagnostic criteria. Semin Arthritis Rheum. 2016;46:319–29.

17. Gultuna S, Tezel N, Ozalp Ates FS. Fibromyalgia in the patients with allergic rhinitis: its prevalence and impact on the quality of life. Am J Rhinol Allergy. 2019;33(6):716–22.
18. Chester AC. Symptoms of rhinosinusitis in patients with unexplained chronic fatigue or bodily pain: a pilot study. Arch Intern Med. 2003;163(15):1832–6.
19. Hamdan AL, Hosri J, Yammine Y, Ghzayel L, Hadi J, Moussawi MA, Romanos M, Nader N, Uthman I. Voice disorders in patients with fibromyalgia: case series and review of the literature. J Voice. 2024; https://doi.org/10.1016/j.jvoice.2024.06.027.
20. Gilheaney Ó, Hussey J, McTiernan K. The lived experiences of oropharyngeal dysphagia in adults living with fibromyalgia. Health Expect. 2024;27(1):e13932.
21. Yunus MB. Towards a model of pathophysiology of fibromyalgia: aberrantcentral pain mechanisms with peripheral modulation [Editorial]. J Rheumatol. 1992;19:846–50.
22. Li J, Simone DA, Larson AA. Windup leads to characteristics of centralsensitization. Pain. 1999;79:75–82.
23. Cook DB, Lange G, Ciccone DS, Liu WC, Steffener J, Natelson BH. Functional imaging of pain in patients with primary fibromyalgia. J Rheumatol. 2004;31:364–78.
24. Gracely RH, Petzke F, Wolf JM, Clauw DJ. Functional magnetic resonanceimaging evidence of augmented pain processing in fibromyalgia. Arthritis Rheum. 2002;46:1333–43.
25. Staud R, Cannon RC, Mauderli AP, et al. Temporal summation of pain from mechanical stimulation of muscletissue in normal controls and subjects with fibromyalgia syndrome. Pain. 2003;102:87–95.
26. Kosek E, Hansson P. Modulatory influence on somatosensory perceptionfrom vibration and heterotopic noxious conditioning stimulation (HNCS) infibromyalgia patients and healthy subjects. Pain. 1997;70:41–51.
27. Suhnan AP, Finch PM, Drummond PD. Hyperacusis in chronic pain: neural interactions between the auditory and nociceptive systems. Int J Audiol. 2017;56(11):801–9.
28. Grayston R, Czanner G, Elhadd K, et al. A systematic review and meta-analysis of the prevalence of small fiber pathology in fibromyalgia: implications for a new paradigm in fibromyalgia etiopathogenesis. Semin Arthritis Rheum. 2019;48(5):933–40.
29. Galosi E, Truini A, Di Stefano G. A systematic review and meta-analysis of the prevalence of small fibre impairment in patients with fibromyalgia. Diagnostics (Basel). 2022;12(5):1135.
30. Goebel A, Krock E, Gentry C, et al. Passive transfer of fibromyalgia symptoms from patients to mice. J Clin Invest. 2021;131(13):e144201.
31. Bazzichi L, Rossi A, Massimetti G, et al. Cytokine patterns in fibromyalgia and their correlation with clinical manifestations. Clin Exp Rheumatol. 2007;25(2):225–30.
32. Bote ME, García JJ, Hinchado MD, Ortega E. Inflammatory/stress feedback dysregulation in women with fibromyalgia. Neuroimmunomodulation. 2012;19(6):343–51.
33. Kadetoff D, Lampa J, Westman M, et al. Evidence of central inflammation in fibromyalgia-increased cerebrospinal fluid interleukin-8 levels. J Neuroimmunol. 2012;242(1–2):33–8.
34. Houvenagel E, Forzy G, Leloire O, Gallois P, Hary S, Hautecoeur P, et al. Cerebrospinal fluid monoamines in primary fibromyalgia. Rev Rhum Mal Osteoartic. 1990;57:21–3.
35. Watkins LR, Milligan ED, Maier SF. Glial activation: a driving force forpathological pain. Trends Neurosci. 2001;24:450–5.
36. Gabuzda D, Wang J. Chemokine receptors and virus entry in the centralnervous system. J Neurovirol. 1999;5:643–58.
37. Rock RB, Gekker G, Hu S, Sheng WS, Cheeran M, Lokensgard JR, Peterson PK. Role of microglia in central nervous system infections. Clin Microbiol Rev. 2004;17(4):942–64.
38. Watkins LR, Maier SF. The pain of being sick: implications of immune-to-brain communication for understanding pain. Annu Rev Psychol. 2000;51:29–57.
39. Watkins LR, Maier SF. Immune regulation of central nervous system functions: from sickness responses to pathological pain. J Intern Med. 2005;257:139–55.
40. Watkins LR, Martin D, Ulrich P, Tracey KJ, Maier SF. Evidence for the involvement of spinal cord glia in subcutaneous formalin induced hyperalgesia in the rat. Pain. 1997;71:225–35.

41. Raghavendra V, Tanga F, DeLeo JA. Inhibition of microglial activation attenuates the development but not existing hypersensitivity in a rat model of neuropathy. J Pharmacol Exp Ther. 2003;306:624–30.
42. Yunus MB, Dailey JW, Aldag JC, Masi AT, Jobe PC. Plasma tryptophan and other amino acids in primary fibromyalgia: a controlled study. J Rheumatol. 1992;19:90–4.
43. Hrycaj P, Stratz T, Mu¨ller W. Platelet 3H-imipramine uptake receptordensity and serum serotonin levels in patients with fibromyalgia/fibrositis syndrome [Letter]. J Rheumatol. 1993;20:1986–8.
44. Wolfe F, Russell IJ, Vipraio G, Ross K, Anderson J. Serotonin levels, pain threshold, and fibromyalgia symptoms in the general population. J Rheumatol. 1997;24:555–9.
45. Russell IJ, Vaeroy H, Javors M, Nyberg F. Cerebrospinal fluid biogenicamine metabolites in fibromyalgia/fibrositis syndrome and rheumatoid arthritis. Arthritis Rheum. 1992;35:550–6.
46. Offenbaecher M, Bondy B, de Jonge S, Glatzeder K, Kru¨ger M, Schoeps P, et al. Possible association of fibromyalgia with a polymorphism in the serotonintransporter gene regulatory region. Arthritis Rheum. 1999;42:2482–8.
47. Cohen H, Buskila D, Neumann L, Ebstein RP. Confirmation of an association between fibromyalgia and serotonin transporter promoter region (5-HTTLPR) polymorphism, and relationship to anxiety-related personality traits [Letter]. Arthritis Rheum. 2002;46:845–7.
48. Gursoy S. Absence of association of the serotonin transporter gene polymorphism with the mentally healthy subset of fibromyalgia patients. Clin Rheumatol. 2002;21:194–7.
49. Wood PB. Stress and dopamine: implications for the pathophysiology of chronic widespread pain. Med Hypotheses. 2004;62:420–4.
50. Malt EA, Olafsson S, Aakvaag A, Lund A, Ursin H. Altered dopamine D2receptor function in fibromyalgia patients: a neuroendocrine study with buspirone in women with fibromyalgia compared to female population based controls. J Affect Disord. 2003;75:77–82.
51. Crofford LJ. The hypothalamic-pituitary-adrenal axis in the pathogenesis of rheumatic diseases. Endocrinol Metab Clin N Am. 2002;31:1–13.
52. Crofford LJ, Pillemer SR, Kalogeras KT, Cash JM, Michelson D, Kling MA, et al. Hypothalamic-pituitary-adrenal axis perturbations in patients with fibromyalgia. Arthritis Rheum. 1994;37:1583–92.
53. Ferraccioli G, Cavalieri F, Salaffi F, Fontana S, Scita F, Nolli M, et al. Neuroendocrinologic findings in primary fibromyalgia (soft tissue chronic painsyndrome) and in other chronic rheumatic conditions (rheumatoid arthritis, lowback pain). J Rheumatol. 1990;17:869–73.
54. Griep EN, Boersma JW, Lentjes EG, Prins AP, van der Korst JK, de KloetER. Function of the hypothalamic-pituitary-adrenal axis in patients with fibro-myalgia and low back pain. J Rheumatol. 1998;25:1374–81.
55. Griep EN, Boersma JW, de Kloet ER. Altered reactivity of the hypothalamic-pituitary-adrenal axis in the primary fibromyalgia syndrome. J Rheumatol. 1993;20:469–74.
56. Carroll BJ, Feinberg M, Greden JF, Tarika J, Albala AA, Haskett RF, et al. A specific laboratory test for the diagnosis of melancholia. Standardization, validation, and clinical utility. Arch Gen Psychiatry. 1981;38:15–22.
57. Bennett RM. Physical fitness and muscle metabolism in the fibromyalgia syndrome: an overview. J Rheumatol Suppl. 1989;19:28–9.
58. Le Goff P. Is fibromyalgia a muscle disorder? Joint Bone Spine. 2006;73(3):239–42.
59. Lund E, Kendall SA, Janerot-Sjøberg B, et al. Muscle metabolism in fibromyalgia studied by P-31 magnetic resonance spectroscopy during aerobic and anaerobic exercise. Scand J Rheumatol. 2003;32(3):138–45.
60. Ruggiero L, Manganelli F, Santoro L. Muscle pain syndromes and fibromyalgia: the role of muscle biopsy. Curr Opin Support Palliat Care. 2018;12(3):382–7.
61. Cordero MD, de Miguel M, Carmona-López I, et al. Oxidative stress and mitochondrial dysfunction in fibromyalgia. Neuro Endocrinol Lett. 2010;31(2):169–73.
62. Beyaztas H, Aktas S, Guler EM, et al. Oxidative stress may be a contributing factor in fibromyalgia patients' pain mechanisms. Reumatismo. 2023;75(3) https://doi.org/10.4081/reumatismo.2023.1550.

63. Neyal M, Yimenicioglu F, Aydeniz A, et al. Plasma nitrite levels, total antioxidant status, total oxidant status, and oxidative stress index in patients with tension-type headache and fibromyalgia. Clin Neurol Neurosurg. 2013;115(6):736–4.
64. Meeus M, Nijs J, Hermans L, et al. The role of mitochondrial dysfunctions due to oxidative and nitrosative stress in the chronic pain or chronic fatigue syndromes and fibromyalgia patients: peripheral and central mechanisms as therapeutic targets? Expert Opin Ther Targets. 2013;17(9):1081–9.
65. Häuser W, Sarzi-Puttini P, Fitzcharles MA. Fibromyalgia syndrome: under-, over-and misdiagnosis. Clin Exp Rheumatol. 2019;37(Suppl 116):90–7.
66. Nugraha B, Karst M, Engeli S, Gutenbrunner C. Brain-derived neurotrophic factor and exercise in fibromyalgia syndrome patients: a mini review. Rheumatol Int. 2012;32:2593–9.
67. Giovengo SL, Russell IJ, Larson AA. Increased concentrations of nerve growth factor in cerebrospinal fluid of patients with fibromyalgia. J Rheumatol. 1999;26:1564–9.
68. Choy EH, Arnold LM, Clauw DJ, Crofford LJ, Glass JM, Simon LS, et al. Content and criterion validity of the preliminary core dataset for clinical trials in fibromyalgia syndrome. J Rheumatol. 2009;36:2330–4.
69. Fitzcharles MA, Boulos P. Inaccuracy in the diagnosis of fibromyalgia syndrome: analysis of referrals. Rheumatology (Oxford). 2003;42:263–7.
70. Wolfe F, Häuser W. Fibromyalgia diagnosis and diagnostic criteria. Ann Med. 2011;43(7):495–502.
71. Wolfe F. New American College of Rheumatology criteria for fibromyalgia: a twenty-year journey. Arthritis Care Res. 2010;62(5):583–4.
72. Wolfe F, Clauw DJ, Fitzcharles MA, Goldenberg DL, Häuser W, Katz RS, Mease P, Russell AS, Russell IJ, Winfield JB. Fibromyalgia criteria and severity scales for clinical and epidemiological studies: a modification of the ACR Preliminary Diagnostic Criteria for Fibromyalgia. J Rheumatol. 2011;38(6):1113–22.
73. Smythe HA. Unhelpful criteria sets for "diagnosis" and "assessment of severity" of fibromyalgia. J Rheumatol. 2011;38:975–8.
74. Arnold LM, Bennett RM, Crofford LJ, Dean LE, Clauw DJ, Goldenberg DL, et al. AAPT diagnostic criteria for fibromyalgia. J Pain. 2019;20:611–28.
75. Salaffi F, Di Carlo M, Farah S, Atzeni F, Buskila D, Ablin JN, et al. Diagnosis of fibromyalgia: comparison of the 2011/2016 ACR and AAPT criteria and validation of the modified Fibromyalgia Assessment Status. Rheumatology (Oxford). 2020;59:3042–9.
76. Arnold LM, Clauw DJ, McCarberg BH. Improving the recognition and diagnosis of fibromyalgia. Mayo Clin Proceed. 2011;86(5):457–64.
77. Buskila D, Cohen H, Neumann L, Ebstein RP. An association between fibromyalgia and the dopamine D4 receptor exon III repeat polymorphism and relationship to novelty seeking personality traits. Mol Psychiatry. 2004;9:730–1.
78. Caccamo D, Cesareo E, Mariani S, Raskovic D, Ientile R, Curro M, Korkina L, De Luca C. Xenobiotic sensor- and metabolism-related gene variants in environmental sensitivity-related illnesses: a survey on the Italian population. Oxidative Med Cell Longev. 2013;2013:831969.
79. Crofford LJ, Pillemer SR, Kalogeras KT, Cash JM, Michelson D, Kling MA, Sternberg EM, Gold PW, Chrousos GP, Wilder RL. Hypothalamic-pituitary-adrenal axis perturbations in patients with fibromyalgia. Arthritis Rheum. 1994;37(11):1583–92.
80. Anderberg UM, Liu Z, Berglund L, Nyberg F. Elevated plasma levels of neuropeptide Y in female fibromyalgia patients. Eur J Pain. 1999;3(1):19–30.
81. Iannuccelli C, Di Franco M, Alessandri C, Guzzo MP, Croia C, Di Sabato F, Foti M, Valesini G. Pathophysiology of fibromyalgia: a comparison with the tension-type headache, a localized pain syndrome. Ann N Y Acad Sci. 2010;1193:78–83.
82. Valdés M, Collado A, Bargalló N, Vázquez M, Rami L, Gómez E, Salamero M. Increased glutamate/glutamine compounds in the brains of patients with fibromyalgia: a magnetic resonance spectroscopy study. Arthritis Rheum. 2010;62(6):1829–36.

83. Sarchielli P, Mancini ML, Floridi A, Coppola F, Rossi C, Nardi K, Acciarresi M, Pini LA, Calabresi P. Increased levels of neurotrophins are not specific for chronic migraine: evidence from primary fibromyalgia syndrome. J Pain. 2007;8(9):737–45.
84. Laske C, Stransky E, Eschweiler GW, Klein R, Wittorf A, Leyhe T, Richartz E, Köhler N, Bartels M, Buchkremer G, Schott K. Increased BDNF serum concentration in fibromyalgia with or without depression or antidepressants. J Psychiatr Res. 2007;41(7):600–5.
85. Bazzichi L, Rossi A, Zirafa C, Monzani F, Tognini S, Dardano A, Santini F, Tonacchera M, De Servi M, Giacomelli C, et al. Thyroid autoimmunity may represent a predisposition for the development of fibromyalgia? Rheumatol Int. 2012;32:335–41.
86. Ciregia F, Giacomelli C, Giusti L, Lucacchini A, Bazzichi L. Diagnosis of fibromyalgia syndrome: potential biomarkers and proteomic approach. IntechOpen; 2011.
87. Klein R, Berg PA. Diagnostic relevance of antibodies to serotonin and phospholipids in fibromyalgia syndrome. J Rheumatol. 2002;29(2):395–6.
88. Bazzichi L, Palego L, Giannaccini G, Rossi A, De Feo F, Giacomelli C, Betti L, Giusti L, Mascia G, Bombardieri S, Lucacchini A. Altered amino acid homeostasis in subjects affected by fibromyalgia. Clin Biochem. 2009;42(10–11):1064–70.
89. Maes M, Verkerk R, Delmeire L, Van Gastel A, van Hunsel F, Scharpe S. Serotonergic markers and lowered plasma branched-chain-amino acid concentrations in fibromyalgia. Psychiatry Res. 2000;97:11–20.

Prevalence of Voice Disorders in Fibromyalgia

5

Abdul-latif Hamdan, Robert Thayer Sataloff,
and Mary J. Hawkshaw

Prevalence of Voice Disorders in Fibromyalgia

As discussed in Chap. 2, the phonatory system consists of a power source, an oscillator, and resonators. The power source energizes the oscillator while the resonators act to amplify and shape the vocal signal [1]. All three components of the phonatory apparatus are linked intricately to the musculoskeletal system. The power supply depends on the diaphragm and external intercostal muscles for inhalation and on the internal intercostals and parasternal muscles for exhalation. Dysfunction in these respiratory muscles can disturb in the expiratory flow with subsequent change in voice quality [2]. Similarly, alteration in the biomechanics of any of the intrinsic laryngeal muscles secondary to metabolic, inflammatory or vascular changes, can lead to dysregulation of pitch and volume control. In addition, change in the length or configuration of the vocal tract secondary to a reduced activity of the strap muscles and/or pharyngeal muscles can result in alteration in the position and distribution of the formant frequencies. The formant frequencies are primarily responsible for the timbre of the voice, a unique feature of the speaker's identity that is determined largely the length and shape of the vocal tract [3].

Despite the strong link between the phonatory system and the musculoskeletal system, little has been written on voice disorders in Fibromyalgia (FM) patients. Fibromyalgia affects the central and peripheral nervous system, as well as skeletal muscles including those related to phonation. In addition to the diffuse, widespread pain, somatic and psychological symptoms, affected patients typically suffer from muscle dysfunction associated with a decrease in muscle strength and endurance which commonly affects the vocal apparatus. In 2013, *Gurbuzler et al.* investigated the subjective changes in voice quality in a cohort of 30 patients with FM and reported higher Vocal Handicap Index-10 (VHI-10) scores in comparison to controls (7.90 ± 7.58 in vs. 1.83 ± 2.82, respectively). The auditory perceptual

A.-l. Hamdan et al., *Voice Disorders in Fibromyalgia*,
https://doi.org/10.1007/978-3-031-97751-0_5

evaluation also revealed a higher mean rating ~~of~~ on GRBAS scale in the diseased group compared to the control group (2.50 ± 1.97 vs. 0.56 ± 1.04, respectively). The voice of FM patients was rated as more strained compared to healthy subjects. The higher rating of the overall grade of dysphonia and that of strain was attributed hypothetically to high tension in the intrinsic laryngeal muscles and to weakness in the cervical muscles responsible for the cephalocaudal movement of the larynx. Despite the high auditory perceptual rating and self-reported vocal handicap score in FM patients, there was no significant difference in the fundamental frequency, noise-to-harmonic ratio, or any of the perturbation parameters measured in comparison to controls. The discrepancy between the subjective voice outcome measures and acoustic findings was attributed to the limited sensitivity of acoustic analysis in capturing all aspects of disease-induced phonatory instability [4]. Other findings in FM patients were the lower voice intensity and shorter maximum phonation time (MPT) in comparison to controls. These were ascribed to respiratory dysfunction, namely the decrease in pulmonary strength and chest wall compliance resulting in diminished expiratory volume and maximum expiratory pressure [5]. In 2020, *Piersiala et al.* investigated the laryngeal manifestations of 215 patients with chronic pain syndromes (CPS), 77 of whom had Fibromyalgia syndrome (FMS), and noted muscle tension dysphonia (MTD) in 30.7% of the cases vs. 17.6% in controls. Patients with CPS were more likely to have functional voice disorders than those with no CPS (OR of 1.74; 95% CI). Patients with FM syndrome were twice as likely to have MTD and three times more likely to have paradoxical vocal fold motion than healthy controls [6]. In 2023, *Basar et al.* conducted a prospective study on the prevalence of dysphonia in a cohort of 25 patients with FM and noted significantly higher visual analog scale (VAS) scores for hoarseness in comparison to 25 healthy controls matched by demographic characteristics. Using acoustic analysis, the authors also found a significantly higher shimmer value and a significantly shorter MPT in the diseased group compared to controls (3.20 ± 1.91 vs. 2.04 ± 0.46, and 14.87 ± 5.23 vs. 17.19 ± 3.32, respectively). The authors attributed these differences to respiratory dysfunction, namely the decrease in expiratory pressure in patients with FM [7]. In 2024, *Hamdan et al.* investigated the prevalence of voice disorders and their impact on quality of life in 35 patients diagnosed with FM and noted a significantly higher mean VHI-10 score in comparison to healthy controls with no FM (8.51 ± 7.66 vs. 0.74 ± 0.98, respectively). More than one third of the study group (37.1%) had a VHI-10 score above 11 vs. none in the control group. Furthermore, there was a positive correlation between the VHI-10 score and the scores of two screening questionnaires for FM, namely the Fibromyalgia Rapid Screening Tool (FiRST) and the short form of the McGill pain questionnaire (SF-MPQ) [8].

The strong link between FM and voice disorders is accompanied by an increased prevalence of swallowing disorders in patients with FM. This is not surprising given the anatomic proximity of the larynx to the pharynx and the strong overlap in neuromuscular structure. Numerous studies have shown that FM patients are at a higher risk of having swallowing symptoms in comparison to normal subjects. In a systematic review of the literature on eating and swallowing problems in patients with FM,

Gilheaney and Chadwick reported dysphagia in 51.9% of the cases, with a wide range from 25.6% to 77.2% [9]. *Rhodus et al.* investigated the prevalence of dysphagia in 67 FM patients and noted a higher prevalence in comparison to controls (37.3% vs. 0.4%, respectively) [10]. *Leon et al.* used the EAT-10 questionnaire to screen for dysphagia in a cohort of Hispanic patients with FM and reported an increased risk in almost two-thirds of their participants [11]. In another cross-sectional study that included 46 women with FM, *Villaverde-Rodriguez et al.* reported dysphagia in 65.21% of the cases, with adverse effect on quality of life in two out of five patients [12]. *Gilheaney et al.* conducted a survey on the type of eating complaints in 1983 FM patients and noted that food sticking in the throat, need to exert extra effort to swallow, and dryness in the mouth were the most common symptoms, the occurrence of which varied from 85–89% of the cases [13].

The high prevalence of voice and swallowing disorders in patients with FM can be attributed to central nervous system dysregulation and to the laryngopharyngeal manifestation of the disease, namely dysfunction in the intrinsic and extrinsic muscles of the larynx and pharynx. There are many suggested etiologies for muscle dysfunction in FM patients including chronic inflammation, metabolic alterations and oxidative stress [14, 15]. The muscle dysfunction may or may be accompanied by alteration in the biomechanics of the laryngeal framework and limitation in its movement. A detailed description of the musculoskeletal manifestation of FM and their impact on voice can be found in Chap. 12 of this book. Other comorbidities that may cause phonatory disorders in FM include reflux disease, breathing impairment, sleep disturbances and body fatigue. The adverse effects of these comorbidities on voice are discussed in Chaps. 8, 9, 14 and 15 of this book.

The Prevalence of FM in Patients with Voice Disorders

Looking at the association of FM and dysphonia from a laryngological perspective numerous studies have shown a high risk for FM in patients with voice disorders. In a review of 153 patients with MTD, *Craig et al.* noted the presence of FM among other co-morbidities such as chronic fatigue syndrome in 8% of their study group, in comparison to a prevalence of 2–4% in the general population [16–18]. The diagnosis of FM was based on review of the medical records. The authors highlighted the added value of physical therapy in selected patients with MTD, and the need for a more holistic approach in the treatment of functional voice disorders [16]. In another study on the prevalence of FM in MTD, *Hamdan et al.* found that patients with MTD were at a higher risk of developing FM in comparison to controls (56% vs. 4%, respectively). Moreover, there was a positive correlation between the Fibromyalgia Rapid Screening Test (FiRST) score and the VHI-10 score (r value 0.39, $p = 0.09$). The mean VHI-10 score was significantly higher in those who screened positive for FM in comparison to those who did not. The authors opined that FM could be a frequent comorbid condition in patients with MTD, and that MTD could be a laryngeal manifestation of FM [19]. The link between MTD and FM was attributed to central nervous system dysregulation that has been reported in both disorders. Central sensitization in Fibromyalgia can lead to complex physiologic disturbances that may affect the phonatory apparatus [20]. That said, the authors concluded that MTD is one additional disorder that could be included in the diagnosis of FM. In another prospective study that included 42 participants, the same authors found that patients with MTD were 6.67 times more likely to have FM in comparison to healthy controls with no history of voice disorders. There was a significant difference in the score of the FiRST between the two subgroups (40% in the diseased group vs. 9.1%, in controls, p value 0.03). The authors stressed the need for a more holistic approach in the management of patients with MTD [8].

In summary, Fibromyalgia increases the risk of voice disorders. These symptoms can be overlooked easily given the complexity of the disease and its multifaceted clinical presentation. Affected patients with voice complaints should be examined to rule out functional and or structural laryngeal disorders. The pathophysiology of dysphonia in FM is far from being understood. Central and peripheral etiologies have been suggested given the neuromuscular structure of the laryngeal framework. The laryngeal manifestation of comorbidities in FM also may contribute to the pathophysiology of dysphonia. Future research using serologic inflammatory and other biomarkers, as well as electromyography of the laryngeal muscles and other studies are needed to improve our understanding of phonatory disorders in FM.

References

1. Hamdan AL, Sataloff RT, Hawkshaw MJ. Anatomy and physiology of the voice. In: Office-based laryngeal surgery. Cham: Springer; 2022. p. 3–14.
2. Jiang J, O'Mara T, Conley D, Hanson D. Phonation threshold pressure measurements during phonation by airflow interruption. Laryngoscope. 1999;109(3):425–32.
3. Sundberg J. Vocal tract resonance. In: Sataloff RT, editor. The professional voice. 4th ed. San Diego: Plural Publishing; 2017. p. 309–29.
4. Gurbuzler L, Inanir A, Yelken K, Koc S, Eyibilen A, Uysal IO. Voice disorder in patients with fibromyalgia. Auris Nasus Larynx. 2013;40(6):554–7.
5. Weiss DJ, Kreck T, Albert RK. Dyspnea resulting from fibromyalgia. Chest. 1998;113(1):246–9.
6. Piersiala K, Akst LM, Hillel AT, Best SR. Chronic pain syndromes and their laryngeal manifestations. JAMA Otolaryngol Head Neck Surg. 2020;146(6):543–9.
7. Basar G, Kaleoglu Aslan O, Surmeli M. Relationship between dysphonia and anxiety in fibromyalgia syndrome. Eur Arch Otorrinolaringol. 2023;280(1):285–8.
8. Hamdan AL, Hosri J, Yammine Y, Ghzayel L, Hadi J, Moussawi MA, Romanos M, Nader N, Uthman I. Voice disorders in patients with fibromyalgia: case series and review of the literature. J Voice. 2024; https://doi.org/10.1016/j.jvoice.2024.06.027.
9. Gilheaney Ó, Chadwick A. The prevalence and nature of eating and swallowing problems in adults with fibromyalgia: a systematic review. Dysphagia. 2024;39(1):92–108.
10. Rhodus NL, Fricton J, Carlson P, Messner R. Oral symptoms associated with fibromyalgia syndrome. J Rheumatol. 2003;30(8):1841–5.
11. Colón León RA, Centeno Vázquez MA. EAT-10 and Hispanics with fibromyalgia. Dysphagia. 2021;36:1118–4.
12. Del Carmen Villaverde-Rodríguez M, Correa-Rodríguez M, Casas-Barragán A, Tapia-Haro RM, Aguilar-Ferrándiz ME. Orofacial pain and risk of dysphagia in women with fibromyalgia: a cross-sectional observational study. Am J Speech Lang Pathol. 2024;33(2):883–92.

13. Gilheaney Ó, Costello C, McTiernan K. Surveying the international prevalence and nature of eating, drinking and swallowing difficulties in adults presenting with fibromyalgia. Dysphagia. 2024;39(3):495–503.
14. Jurado-Priego LN, Cueto-Urena C, Ramirez-Exposito MJ, Martinez-Martos JM. Fibromyalgia: a review of the pathophysiological mechanisms and multidisciplinary treatment strategies. Biomedicines. 2024;12(7):1543.
15. Siracusa R, Di Paola R, Cuzzocrea S, Impellizzeri D. Fibromyalgia: Pathogenesis, mechanisms, diagnosis and treatment options update. Int J Mol Sci. 2021;22(8):3891.
16. Craig J, Tomlinson C, Stevens K, Kotagal K, Fornadley J, Jacobson B, Garrett CG, Francis DO. Combining voice therapy and physical therapy: a novel approach to treating muscle tension dysphonia. J Commun Disord. 2015;58:169–78.
17. Berwick R, Barker C, Goebel A, Guideline Development Group. The diagnosis of fibromyalgia syndrome. Clin Med (Lond). 2022;22(6):570–4.
18. Cabo-Meseguer A, Cerdá-Olmedo G, Trillo-Mata JL. Fibromyalgia: prevalence, epidemiologic profiles and economic costs. Med Clin (Barc). 2017;149(10):441–8. English, Spanish.
19. Hamdan AL, Alam E, Feghali PAR, Fadel C, Jabbour C, Ghanem A. Risk of fibromyalgia in patients with primary muscle tension dysphonia: a possible local manifestation of a musculoskeletal systemic disorder. J Laryngol Otol. 2024;138(3):341–4.
20. Sarzi Puttini P, Atzeni F, Di Franco M, Buskila D, Alciati A, Giacomelli C, Rossi A, Bazzichi L. Dysfunctional syndromes and fibromyalgia: a 2012 critical digest. Clin Exp Rheumatol. 2012;30(74):S143–51.

6 Breathing Disorders in Fibromyalgia: Is the Power Source of Voice in Jeopardy

Abdul-latif Hamdan, Robert Thayer Sataloff, and Mary J. Hawkshaw

Respiratory Dysfunction in Fibromyalgia

Respiratory dysfunction is a known co-morbidity in Fibromyalgia (FM). Among the most common symptoms are dyspnea and change in breathing pattern. The prevalence of respiratory symptoms varies between studies based on the severity of the disease and associated co-morbidities. *Caidahl et al.* investigated 87 women with chronic primary FM and noted dyspnea in 84% of the cases. There was also a positive correlation between the grade of dyspnea and breathing rate at rest [1]. In a study in which dyspnea was induced gradually by increasing ventilation and carbon dioxide (CO_2) pressure, *Van Den Houte et al.* found that FM patients had significantly more dyspnea in the recovery phase compared to healthy controls. The dyspnea was explained on the basis of functional somatic symptoms which were more prevalent in the diseased group [2]. The respiratory symptoms in FM often overlap with symptoms of other chronic respiratory diseases, thus masking the diagnosis and at times worsening the treatment outcome. *Hyland et al.* compared the symptoms of FM with the extra-pulmonary symptoms of asthma in 100 patients who had been diagnosed with severe asthma and noted a similarity index of 0.75. The similarity index was computed by examining the overlap in symptoms with 0 indicating no relationship and one indicating an identical symptom patterns. The authors highlighted the strong similarity between the extra-pulmonary symptoms of asthma and FM, and they stressed the need for a holistic approach in the management of patients with pulmonary symptoms [3]. *Martinez-Moragon et al.* investigated the impact of FM on asthma control in a group of patients (n = 56) with asthma and FM in comparison to another group with asthma and no FM (n = 36). The results indicated lower scores for asthma control and asthma-related quality of life, and worse perception of dyspnea in those with

A.-l. Hamdan et al., *Voice Disorders in Fibromyalgia*,
https://doi.org/10.1007/978-3-031-97751-0_6

co-existent FM. Furthermore, patients with FM had a higher prevalence of anxiety and depression using the Hospital Anxiety and Depression Scale (HADS) in comparison to those with no FM [4].

Respiratory symptoms in FM may coexist with chest pain. Affected patients can present with or complain of chest pain during the course of their disease. *Weiss et al.* reported two cases of intermittent dyspnea associated with chest wall pain who were investigated extensively for upper and lower airway diseases with no clear diagnosis. Upon further review and closer examination, their dyspnea was attributed to FM. Both patients improved after being treated for their primary condition [5]. Wise et al. reviewed the causes of non-cardiac chest wall pain in 100 patients and noted FM as a cause in 5% of the cases. Musculoskeletal chest wall syndrome was considered as one of the many musculoskeletal manifestations of FM [6].

It is important to note that respiratory symptoms in FM can lead to a decrease in physical activity and exercise tolerance in affected patients. In 2011, *Homann et al.* compared the functional capacity of 19 women with FM to 20 healthy controls using the 6-Min walk test (6-MWT) and found that those with FM walked a significantly shorter distance in comparison to those with no FM (473.52 ± 77.84 m vs. 541.75 ± 85.62 m, respectively). Moreover, there was a negative correlation between the 6-MWT score, the Fibromyalgia Impact Questionnaire score and the Health Assessment Questionnaire score [7]. Similarly, in 2014, *Roman et al.* evaluated the performance of 36 women with FM using the 6-MWT and noted that they covered a shorter distance and had a lower cardiorespiratory response in comparison to healthy controls [8].

Possible Causes of Respiratory Symptoms in FM

The causes of respiratory symptoms in FM have been investigated by numerous authors using spirometry and other electrophysiologic tests such as electromyography and chest wall expansion measures with no clear understanding of the exact pathophysiology [1]. In 1990, *Lurie et al.* investigated the respiratory function of 87 women with chronic primary FM and found significantly lower maximum inspiratory pressure (MIP) and maximum expiratory pressure (MEP) in comparison to 61 healthy controls. These findings were ascribed to dysfunction in the respiratory muscles, particularly the diaphragm [9]. In 2004, *Sahin et al.* investigated pulmonary muscle strength in a cohort of female patients diagnosed with FM and also noted a decrease in MIP and MEP in comparison to healthy controls matched by age, gender and body mass Index. Moreover, both MIP and MEP correlated significantly with handgrip strength which was measured using the Jamar handheld dynamometer (Fabrication Enterprises, Elmsford, NY) [10]. In 2016, *Rizzi et al.* reported a significant difference in the carbon monoxide diffusing capacity, alveolar-capillary membrane and pulmonary capillary blood volume in patients with FM in comparison to healthy controls. Moreover, there was a significant correlation between those variables and the COMPASS-31 score, Visual Analog Scale (VAS) score for pain and the Raynaud's Condition Score (RCS), a scale commonly used assess the level of difficulty patients experience due to Raynaud's phenomenon [11]. In 2016, *Forti et al.* investigated the pulmonary function and respiratory muscle strength in a cohort of 23 patients with FM and found significantly lower maximum voluntary ventilation and MIP in comparison to controls [12]. In 2023, *Cuenca-Martinez* conducted a review on respiratory function in patients with chronic pain and found that those with FM exhibited a decrease in maximal voluntary ventilation (MVV) in comparison to healthy subjects [13]. In 2024, *Jonsson et al.* investigated acid-base imbalance as an indicator of respiratory dysfunction in 36 women with FM and noted significantly lower levels compared to healthy controls. Moreover, there was a significantly higher level of lactate in the diseased group. The authors suggested that most of their findings were secondary to compensatory chronic hyperventilation [14].

In many studies, the decrease in maximum respiratory pressures in FM patients has been associated with a decrease in chest wall compliance. In 2002, *Ozgocmen et al.* reported a decrease in chest expansion and respiratory muscle strength in 30 female patients with FM in comparison to healthy controls. There was a significant positive correlation between chest expansion and MIP ($r = 0.49$) and MEP ($r = 0.57$). Although one third of the study group had chest pain, there was no significant difference in MIP and MEP between those with or without chest pain. In conclusion, the authors highlighted the possible use of chest expansion as an indicator of respiratory function in patients with FM [15]. In 2016, *Forti et al*, in their study on thoraco-abdominal wall mobility. In FM, patients noted a correlation between MIP and axillary cirtometry which was also significantly lower in comparison to controls. Cirtometry is a valid and reliable method used to measure the circumference of the abdomen and chest during respiration [12]. In 2004, *Sahin et al.* examined pulmonary muscle strength using chest expansion among other measures in 41 women diagnosed with FM syndrome and found no significant difference in comparison to controls, although the dyspnea score was higher in FM patients [16].

In summary, patients with FM suffer from many respiratory symptoms such as dyspnea, abnormal respiratory pattern, and chest pain. These symptoms are more often than not associated with normal pulmonary function testing except for a decrease in maximum respiratory pressures, decrease in maximum voluntary ventilation and a decrease in chest wall expansion. The respiratory symptoms of FM also may coincide with symptoms of other respiratory diseases thus worsening the clinical presentation of affected patients and at times jeopardizing the control of their disease. Proper awareness of the respiratory symptoms of FM and early diagnosis of comorbid respiratory diseases are crucial to optimize treatment. Fibromyalgia should be included in the differential diagnosis of dyspnea particularly in patients with other somatic symptoms.

Impact of Respiratory Dysfunction in Fibromyalgia on Voice

Breathing provides the power source for phonation. The main respiratory muscles are the diaphragm, the intercostal muscles, the abdominal and back muscles [17]. Dysfunction in any of those respiratory muscles can affects phonation. In the section below, the authors suggest several mechanisms through which respiratory dysfunction in FM can impact voice.

Decrease in Lung Function, the Power Source for Phonation

The decrease in lung function in FM patients has been well documented by numerous authors as indicated in the first section of this chapter [10]. The reduction in maximal voluntary ventilation and in maximum respiratory pressures in FM patients in comparison to controls has been attributed to impairment in the activity of the diaphragm in addition to other respiratory muscles. The diaphragm is an important inspiratory respiratory muscle accounting for two-thirds of change in lung volume during quiet breathing. Its movement is linked closely to posture, flexibility of the lower back, and free movement of the abdominal wall [17]. Numerous studies showed that the diaphragm also plays a significant role in stabilizing the vocal tract during phonation [18, 19]. The activity of the diaphragm helps modulate the effect of passive recoil of the intrathoracic structures during exhalation which may not be useful to the speaker. In singers, the function of the diaphragm is even more important. The diaphragm plays a vital role in regulating the subglottic pressure required to sustain a pitch and loudness and to transition between registers. *Leanderson et al.* noted that singers activate the diaphragm in an abrupt manner while sliding down an octave or during the transition from a loud to a soft note [19]. Adjustments in subglottic pressure are attributed to differential contraction of the diaphragm while singing different notes [20]. *Traser et al.* investigated the respiratory dynamics in six professional singers using magnetic resonance imaging (MRI) and noted that there was more than one functional unit in the diaphragm that operate during the emission of different pitches or loudness [21].

Impairment of diaphragm activity produces adverse effects on voice, particularly on the professional voice. A decrease in MIP and MEP secondary to dysfunction in the activity of the diaphragm and other respiratory muscles (intercostal, abdominal and back) in FM undoubtedly impair the ability of singers to perform particularly when they are challenged to use their maximum breathing capacity in vocally demanding tasks.

Decrease in Chest Wall Compliance in FM

Another possible cause for the increased risk for voice disorders in FM is reduced chest wall compliance. Numerous studies indicate that FM patients have a decrease in rib cage movement in comparison to healthy controls [15]. Chest wall movement is of paramount importance in speech and singing. During inhalation, chest wall movement facilitates expansion by contracting the external intercostal muscles, while during exhalation it helps regulate the subglottic pressure by contracting the internal intercostal muscles. Rib cage compliance also assists in providing a steady airflow for phonation [22, 23]. In singing, movement of the chest wall is of greater importance, particularly in singers who rely on costal breathing that focuses on rib cage expansion [24]. *Watson and Hixon* investigated the changes in rib cage dimensions, namely antero-posterior changes during speaking and singing activities in six well trained baritone singers and noted the prominent role of the rib cage in regulating pressure and flow during phonation [25]. In a study on respiratory kinematics and subglottic pressure during pitch jumps, *Traser et al.* noted the parallel movement of the rib cage with the anterior part of the diaphragm during expiration, although the rib cage was not involved in short-term adaptations during rapid pitch jumps [20]. *Binazzi et al.* used non-invasive optoelectronic plethysmography to assess chest wall kinematics during reading and singing in 16 Italian participants and noted that all three different chest components (abdomen apposed to rib cage, lung apposed to rib cage, and abdomen) contributed to the expired volume [26].

A decrease in chest wall compliance in FM undoubtedly limits the ability of the speaker or singer to project his or her voice. The effect is felt more in singers who rely on rib cage pressure-generating capacity to control singing [27]. Dysfunction in the external intercostals in FM patients may affect the fall in pleural pressure and lung expansion during inspiration, whereas dysfunction in the internal interosseous intercostals and triangularis sterni muscles may limit ~~the~~ contraction of the rib cage and the expiratory breathing forces [17, 28]. *Thomasson and Sundberg* investigated inhalation respiratory patterns in five professional singers and found a high consistency between rib cage movement and lung volume change in all the participants. The authors concluded that rib cage movement, in addition to abdominal wall movement, contributes to inhalation breathing during singing [29]. In FM patients, these important actions are compromised leading to impaired support and often compensatory muscle tension dysphonia (MTD).

Restricted Movement and Alteration in Position of the Larynx

Respiratory dysfunction in FM also may affect phonation by impairing the position and movement of the larynx. It is well known that lung volume is an important determinant of the cephalo-caudal position the laryngeal framework and its movement during respiration. Low-lung volume can lead to a high-positioned larynx which may be associated with hard glottal attacks, whereas a high-lung volume is associated with a low-positioned larynx and soft glottal attack [30]. In a study that included 24 subjects who were asked to phonate at different levels of loudness and pitch, *Iwarsson et al.* noted that a decrease in lung volume resulted in an increase in closed quotient and a decrease in glottal leakage [31]. *Sandnes et al.* investigated the impact of inspiratory muscle training on vocal fold motion in 20 healthy volunteers and found that 90% of the participants had laryngeal abduction when the mouth pressure reached 60–80% of the maximal attainable inspiratory mouth pressure [32]. The authors highlighted the added value of inspiratory muscle training in patients with vocal fold dysfunction. Hence, a decrease in respiratory capacity in FM can have adverse effects on the position and movement of the larynx, which in turn may increase laryngeal tension and thus increase the risk dysphonia. This hypothesis remains unproven. Future studies using subjective and objective measures such as electromyography of the strap muscles and dynamic MRI of the larynx and neck are needed to establish the impact of FM on laryngeal movement and position of the laryngeal framework in the neck.

Chest Pain in FM and the "Musculoskeletal Chest Wall Syndrome"

Chest pain is common in FM. A musculoskeletal origin has been suggested as a source of chest pain in 5–20% of patients presenting to the emergency room [10]. The innervation of the chest wall muscles is intimately linked to that of the cervical region through a complex network which includes the intercostal nerves [33, 34]. As such, chest pain may radiate to the neck, and cervical pain may be perceived by the patient as a chest pain. An example is cervico-thoracic angina reported by patients with cardiac diseases who present with neck and jaw pain [35]. Thus, it appears that chest pain in FM can radiate to the neck and impact the function of the laryngeal muscles. Neck pain may limit activity of the cervical muscles imbalance in laryngeal biomechanics, increased tension and increase risk for voice disorders [36]. An analogous example is the adverse effect of musculoskeletal chest injury on voice reported in athletes, often referred to as "musculoskeletal chest wall syndrome" [37].

In summary, breathing disorders in FM secondary to decrease in diaphragm and other respiratory muscle activity and/or chest wall compliance can affect voice by jeopardizing the power source of phonation. The position and movement of the larynx in the neck are also at risk in those with marked breathing impairment. In singing, subtle changes in the ability to modulate subglottic pressure and expiratory flow may limit the ability of a singer to sustain a note or transition between registers. Chest pain in FM may radiate to the neck and causes imbalance in the activity of the laryngeal muscles. Future studies are needed to confirm these suggested mechanisms.

References

1. Caidahl K, Lurie M, Bake B, Johansson G, Wetterqvist H. Dyspnoea in chronic primary fibromyalgia. J Intern Med. 1989;226(4):265–70.
2. Van Den Houte M, Bogaerts K, Van Diest I, De Bie J, Persoons P, Van Oudenhove L, Van den Bergh O. Perception of induced dyspnea in fibromyalgia and chronic fatigue syndrome. J Psychosom Res. 2018;106:49–55.
3. Hyland ME, Lanario JW, Wei Y, Jones RC, Masoli M. Evidence for similarity in symptoms and mechanism: the extra-pulmonary symptoms of severe asthma and the polysymptomatic presentation of fibromyalgia. Immun Inflamm Dis. 2019;7(4):239–49.

4. Martinez-Moragon E, Plaza V, Torres I, Rosado A, Urrutia I, Casas X, Hinojosa B, Blanco-Aparicio M, Delgado J, Quirce S, Sabadell C. Fibromyalgia as a cause of uncontrolled asthma: a case–control multicenter study. Curr Med Res Opin. 2017;33(12):2181–6.
5. Weiss DJ, Kreck T, Albert RK. Dyspnea resulting from fibromyalgia. Chest. 1998;113(1):246–9.
6. Wise CM, Semble EL, Dalton CB. Musculoskeletal chest wall syndromes in patients with noncardiac chest pain: a study of 100 patients. Arch Phys Med Rehabil. 1992;73(2):147–9.
7. Homann D, Stefanello JM, Góes SM, Leite N. Impaired functional capacity and exacerbation of pain and exertion during the 6-minute walk test in women with fibromyalgia. Rev Bras Fisioter. 2011;15(6):474–80. English, Portuguese.
8. Latorre-Román P, Santos-Campos M, Heredia-Jimenez J, Delgado-Fernandez M, Soto-Hermoso V. Analysis of the performance of women with fibromyalgia in the six-minute walk test and its relation with health and quality of life. J Sports Med Phys Fitness. 2014;54(4):511–7.
9. Lurie M, Caidahl K, Johansson G, Bake B. Respiratory function in chronic primary fibromyalgia. Scand J Rehabil Med. 1990;22(3):151–5.
10. Sahin G, Ulubaş B, Calikoğlu M, Bolgen Cime O, Erdoğan C. Is chest expansion a determinant of pulmonary muscle strength in primary fibromyalgia? Joint Bone Spine. 2004;71(2):140–3.
11. Rizzi M, Atzeni F, Airoldi A, Masala IF, Frassanito F, Salaffi F, Macaluso C, Sarzi-Puttini P. Impaired lung transfer factor in fibromyalgia syndrome. Clin Exp Rheumatol. 2016;34(Suppl 96):S114–9.
12. Forti M, Zamunér AR, Andrade CP, Silva E. Lung function, respiratory muscle strength, and thoracoabdominal mobility in women with fibromyalgia syndrome. Respir Care. 2016;61(10):1384–90.
13. Cuenca-Martínez F, Sempere-Rubio N, Muñoz-Gómez E, Mollà-Casanova S, Carrasco-González E, Martínez-Arnau FM. Respiratory function analysis in patients with chronic pain: an umbrella review and meta-analysis of pooled findings. Healthcare (Basel). 2023;11(9):1358.
14. Jonsson K, Pikwer A, Olsson EMG, Peterson M. Hypocapnia in women with fibromyalgia. Scand. J Pain. 2024;24(1) https://doi.org/10.1515/sjpain-2024-0003.
15. Ozgocmen S, Cimen OB, Ardicoglu O. Relationship between chest expansion and respiratory muscle strength in patients with primary fibromyalgia. Clin Rheumatol. 2002;21:19–22.
16. Sahin G, Ulubaş B, Calikoğlu M, Erdoğan C. Handgrip strength, pulmonary function tests, and pulmonary muscle strength in fibromyalgia syndrome: is there any relationship? South Med J. 2004;97(1):25–9.
17. De Troyer A, Boriek AM. Mechanics of the respiratory muscles. Compr Physiol. 2011;1(3):1273–300.
18. De Troyer A, Estenne M. Coordination between rib cage muscles and diaphragm during quiet breathing in humans. J Appl Physiol Respir Environ Exerc Physiol. 1984;57(3):899–906.
19. Leanderson R, Sundberg J, von Euler C. Role of diaphragmatic activity during singing: a study of transdiaphragmatic pressures. J Appl Physiol (1985). 1987;62(1):259–70.
20. Traser L, Burk F, Özen AC, Burdumy M, Bock M, Blaser D, Richter B, Echternach M. Respiratory kinematics and the regulation of subglottic pressure for phonation of pitch jumps: a dynamic MRI study. PLoS One. 2020;15(12):e0244539.
21. Traser L, Özen AC, Burk F, Burdumy M, Bock M, Richter B, Echternach M. Respiratory dynamics in phonation and breathing—a real-time MRI study. Respir Physiol Neurobiol. 2017;236:69–77.
22. Allen W. Breathing in singing. In: Welch G, editor. The Oxford handbook of singing. New York: Oxford Library of Psychology; 2014. p. 87–108.
23. Sundberg J. Breathing behavior during singing. J Sing. 1993;49(4–9):49–51.
24. Vennard W. Singing: the mechanism and the technic. Carl Fischer; 1968.
25. Watson PJ, Hixon TJ. Respiratory kinematics in classical (opera) singers. J Speech Lang Hear Res. 1985;28(1):104–22.
26. Binazzi B, Lanini B, Bianchi R, Romagnoli I, Nerini M, Gigliotti F, Duranti R, Milic-Emili J, Scano G. Breathing pattern and kinematics in normal subjects during speech, singing and loud whispering. Acta Physiol (Oxf). 2006;186(3):233–46.

27. Salomoni S, van den Hoorn W, Hodges P. Breathing and singing: objective characterization of breathing patterns in classical singers. PLoS One. 2016;11(5):e0155084.
28. Han JN, Gayan-Ramirez G, Dekhuijzen R, Decramer M. Respiratory function of the rib cage muscles. Eur Respir J. 1993;6(5):722–8.
29. Thomasson M, Sundberg J. Consistency of inhalatory breathing patterns in professional operatic singers. J Voice. 2001;15(3):373–83.
30. Iwarsson J, Sundberg J. Effects of lung volume on vertical larynx position during phonation. J Voice. 1998;12(2):159–65.
31. Iwarsson J, Thomasson M, Sundberg J. Effects of lung volume on the glottal voice source. J Voice. 1998;12(4):424–33.
32. Sandnes A, Andersen T, Hilland M, Ellingsen TA, Halvorsen T, Heimdal JH, Røksund OD. Laryngeal movements during inspiratory muscle training in healthy subjects. J Voice. 2013;27(4):448–53.
33. Knockaert DC, Buntinx F, Stoens N, Bruyninckx R, Delooz H. Chest pain in the emergency department: the broad spectrum of causes. Eur J Emerg Med. 2002;9(1):25–30.
34. Spalding L, Reay E, Kelly C. Cause and outcome of atypical chest pain in patients admitted to hospital. J R Soc Med. 2003;96(3):122–5.
35. Fam AG, Smythe HA. Musculoskeletal chest wall pain. Can Med Assoc J. 1985;133(5):379.
36. Jain AK, Carruthers BM, Van De Sande MI, et al. Fibromyalgia syndrome: canadian clinical working case definition, diagnostic and treatment protocols–a consensus document. J Musculoskeletal Pain. 2003;11(4):3–107.
37. Winzenberg T, Jones G, Callisaya M. Musculoskeletal chest wall pain. Aust Fam Physician. 2015;44(8):540–4.

Gastro-Intestinal Disorders in Fibromyalgia and Their Impact on Voice

7

Abdul-latif Hamdan, Robert Thayer Sataloff, and Mary J. Hawkshaw

There are numerous studies in the literature on the high prevalence of gastrointestinal (GI) disorders in Fibromyalgia (FM). In 1981, *Yunus et al.* was the first to postulate the link between the gastro-intestinal system and FM [1]. In their detailed study on comorbidities in patients with FM, the prevalence of irritable bowel syndrome (IBS) was noted in 34% of the cases. The authors stressed the need to consider non-musculoskeletal complaints in the evaluation of affected patients [1]. A decade later, *Triadafilopoulos et al.* investigated GI-related symptoms in 123 FM patients and noted a prevalence of 64%. The most common symptoms were abdominal gas and nausea in 59% and 21% of the cases, respectively [2]. Since then, there has been ubiquity of reports in the literature exploring the GI dimension of FM, looking at either GI-related symptoms or GI-related disorders such irritable bowel syndrome (IBS), inflammatory bowel disease (IBD) and gastro-esophageal reflux disease (GERD) [3, 4]. In 2020, in a systematic review on the link between FM and functional gastro-intestinal disorders (FGID), *Erdrich et al.* highlighted the high prevalence of bloating, abdominal pain and IBS in FM patients. The authors reiterated the need to manage GI-related disorders and symptoms in order to improve treatment outcome and overall quality of life of affected patients [4].

Understanding the association between GI disorders and FM is complex. The link between the two has been a subject of thorough investigation in the literature. Several hypotheses were suggested; One is the presence of a common precipitating factor, namely stress. Several studies indicate that stress, a cardinal predisposing factor to FM, can lead to an increase in gastrointestinal secretions, alteration in gut mobility, and to a decrease in the regenerative capacity of the gut mucosal lining. These alterations act to induce and exacerbate GI-related symptoms and disorders [5]. A second possible explanation for the association between FM and GI disorders is the psychosocial state of affected patients. In a study using the Gottschalk-Gleser content analysis method, *Malt et al.* reported the highest score on mutilation anxiety in FM patients and the highest score on death anxiety in patients with functional dyspepsia in comparison to healthy controls. The authors

A.-l. Hamdan et al., *Voice Disorders in Fibromyalgia*,
https://doi.org/10.1007/978-3-031-97751-0_7

noted that anxiety could be a psychological predictor of a neurobiological disturbance in FM [6]. Numerous other reports also asserted the strong link between GI disorders and psychological diseases. In a study on the prevalence of anxiety, depression, and their impact on quality of life in Korean patients with IBS, *Cho HS et al.* found that 38.6% of the study group had experienced anxiety and 38.6% had suffered from depression. These figures were significantly higher than those reported in healthy subjects, namely 24.2% and 16.5% ($p < 0.05$ for both) [7]. Similarly, in a systematic review and meta-analysis on the prevalence of anxiety and depression in patients with IBD, *Barberio B et al.* reported that 38.9% and 57.6% of patients with active IBD experienced anxiety symptoms and depression, respectively, compared to 38.1% and 24.2% in patients with inactive disease [8]. The third possible explanation for the association between GI disorders and FM is the link between the gut and central nervous system, often referred to as the "gut-brain interaction". According to the gut-brain axis, there is a communication between the gut and the central nervous system. The enteric nervous system plays a role in modulating the release of cytokines and neurotransmitters peripherally and centrally thus affecting pain sensitivity [9, 10]. In patients with reflux disease, the retrograde movement of gastric contents into the esophagus stimulates esophageal nociceptors which in turn trigger impulses into the central nervous system. Those nociceptive impulses lead to further increase in pain sensitivity and central sensitization. That said, the increased prevalence of FM in patients with GI disorders can be ascribed mostly to alteration pain processing and central sensitization [9, 11]. The unifying concept on visceral hypersensitivity supports the presence of a systemic etiology for gastro-intestinal disorders and FM.

In this chapter, the authors review the link between FM and three common GI disorders, namely IBS, IBD, and GERD. A thorough discussion on the adverse impact of these GI disorders in FM patients on voice is presented.

The Link Between IBS and FM

Irritable bowel syndrome is a functional disorder that affects 10–20% of the population worldwide with women being affected more than men [12]. This syndrome has adverse effects on quality of life most important of is the psychosocial element [13]. Irritable Bowel syndrome is characterized by a cluster of symptoms that include bloating, abdominal pain, diarrhea and constipation among others. There is no clear understanding of the pathophysiology of this disorder. Suggested aetiologies include alteration in bowel mobility, alteration in visceral sensation and microbiome, disturbance in the immune system and psychological illnesses [2–4]. Other suggested mechanisms include alteration in the afferent visceral signals and central sensitization [14, 15]. *Sivri et al.* investigated symptoms of bowel dysfunction suggestive of IBS in 75 patients with FM and noted a higher prevalence of these symptoms in comparison to controls (41.8% vs. 16%, respectively). The authors opined a common pathophysiology between IBS and FM [5]. In a study investigating the prevalence of FM in a cohort of 1233 patients, *Lee et al.* reported IBS in 21.8% of those with FM. The authors reiterated the strong link between GI-related symptoms in FM patients [16]. *Triadafilopoulos et al.* investigated the prevalence of bowel dysfunction in 123 patients with FM in comparison to 46 normal subjects. Using a validated questionnaire, the authors showed that 73% of those with FM had bowel dysfunction versus none in the control group. The most common bowel-related symptoms were abdominal gas and nausea in 59% and 21% of the cases, respectively. Stress-related abdominal pain was also present in 64% of FM patients [2].

The Impact of IBS in FM Patients on Voice

There are no studies in the literature on voice disorders in FM patients with IBS. However, there are many reports on mental illnesses in IBS and their adverse effect on voice. *Fond et al.* conducted a systematic review of the literature on psychological disorders in IBS and noted a higher prevalence of anxiety and depression in comparison to controls. The authors highlighted the role of psychological illnesses in moderating the frequency and severity of GI symptoms in IBS patients [17]. *Diao et al.* investigated the causal association between psychological factors and IBS using published genome-wide association databases and found that anxiety and depression were among the underlying aetiologies of IBS, with odds ratio of 1.53 and 1.31, 95% CI, respectively [18]. On another note, it is well established in the literature that the psychological state influences voice and that patients with mental illnesses have distinctive voice characteristics. In a study on the correlation between anxiety, depression and vocal handicap in 620 patients with benign dysphonia, *Enin et al.* reported the prevalence of pre-existing anxiety and depression in 20% and 10% of the cases, respectively. The authors also found that those with depression had worse VHI-10 scores than those without anxiety and depression [19]. In a review of 205 patients with benign lesions of the vocal folds, *Makismovic et al.* reported the prevalence of mild-to-severe anxiety in 97.1% of the cases, and mild-to-severe depression in 38.6% of the cases [20]. In a cross-sectional study on the link between psychological distress and voice disorders, *Montgomery et al.* reported a strong correlation between the Hospital Anxiety and Depression scale (HADS) score and emotional VoiSS score. The study included 177 patients, 54.2% of whom had functional dysphonia [21].

In summary, IBS is a common disorder in FM. Symptoms like abdominal pain, bloating, change in bowel habits and others can be added to the armamentarium of somatic complaints in FM. The psychological state of FM patients with IBS may be a risk factor for voice disorders given the high prevalence of psychological illnesses in IBS, and the strong link between voice disorders and the psychological state of affected patients.

The Link Between IBD and FM

Inflammatory bowel disease (IBD) is a chronic inflammatory disorder affecting the gut and other organs in the body leading to an array of symptoms. The most commonly reported conditions are Crohn s disease (CD) and Ulcerative colitis (UC). The pathophysiology of IBD is complex. Both host and environment-related factors act in concert to trigger a inflammatory response often leading to tissue damage. Genetic polymorphism with involvement of the NOD2 and IL12/IL123 complex, and dysregulation in the immune system are the most popular suggested mechanisms [22]. Dietary changes and alteration in gut microbiome may also play a role in the pathogenesis of this disease [22–24]. What is important to note is that IBD is not limited to the gut and that other structures in the body may be involved. Numerous authors highlighted the increased risk of FM in patients with IBD. This is not surprising given the frequent musculoskeletal symptoms in IBD patients often attributed to disease-induced myopathy, osteopenia and osteonecrosis [22]. In 2018, *Chen et al.* investigated the risk of FM in IBD patients using the Taiwan National Health Insurance Research Database (NHIRD) that included 4519 patients. The results showed an adjusted hazard ratio (HR) of 1.70, 95% Confidence Interval. Moreover, male patients and young patients with IBD were found to be at a higher risk of having FM than female patients and elderly. The corresponding adjusted HRs were 2.0 and 1.92, respectively [25]. In 2020, *Buskila et al.* investigated the prevalence of FM in113 patients with IBD and noted that 30% of the participants had FM. Fibromyalgia was more prevalent in patients with CD in comparison to patients with UC and controls. Additionally, CD patients had worse symptoms and higher tender point counts compared to UC patients and healthy subjects. The authors highlighted the need to recognize FM as a comorbidity in patients with IBD [26]. Looking at the other side of the coin, IBD is also a common disease in FM patients. In 2019, *Greebaum et al.* investigated the association between Fibromyalgia, endometriosis and autoimmune diseases and noted a higher prevalence of IBD among other diseases such as SLE and Sjogren in FM patients. Around 6.2% of patients with FM and endometriosis were diagnosed with IBD in comparison to 1% in the control group [27].

The Impact of IBD in FM Patients on Voice

Inflammatory bowel disease is chronic inflammatory condition that targets all organs in the body including the larynx. Affected patients usually present with hoarseness, dysphagia, odynophagia cough and difficulty in breathing. The respiratory symptoms may be subtle initially but can quickly evolve leading to stridor and respiratory distress. In 1994, *Rickli et al.* described a case of UC who presented with a change in voice quality and cough followed by dyspnea and respiratory distress. On laryngeal examination she had severe glottic narrowing secondary to extensive edema. The patient was started on systemic steroids and her symptoms improved gradually. The authors highlighted the infrequent involvement of the larynx in UC

[28]. In 2009, *Hasegawa et al.* reported a 31-year-old-women with a history of GI symptoms suggestive of CD who presented with hoarseness and sore throat in addition to odynophagia. Her symptoms were attributed to focal ulceration of the vocal folds, in the absence of diffuse edema that is commonly seen in CD patients with laryngeal involvement [29]. In 2019, *Loos et al.* reported a 23-year-old-women who presented to the ear, nose and throat (ENT) clinic with hoarseness, dysphagia, odynophagia and stridor. Laryngeal examination showed thickening and fibrosis of the epiglottis with edema of the arytenoids and vocal fold nodules. Biopsy taken from the epiglottis showed signs of chronic inflammation without granuloma. Further review of her medical history revealed symptoms of bloody diarrhea. Rheumatologic investigation was suggestive of UC for which the patient was started on mesalazine [30]. In 2024, *Tahir et al.* conducted a prospective study on vocal symptoms in 28 patients with UC and 22 patients with CD. All patients were evaluated using both subjective and objective voice outcome measures. Patients with UC and CD had higher VHI-10 scores, higher auditory perceptual ratings and significantly higher jitter and shimmer in comparison to controls [31].

In summary, the link between FM and IBD is bidirectional. There are limited case reports on laryngeal involvement in IBD. Suggested mechanisms include alteration in the inflammatory and autoimmune cascades leading to tissue damage. Despite the larynx being a rare target in IBD, FM patients with IBD are at higher risk of having voice disorders given the systemic nature of the disease.

The Link Between GERD and FM

Gastro-esophageal reflux is a common disease affecting millions of people in the United States and 15–40% of adults in Western Europe [32–37]. It is a pathologic condition characterized by retrograde movement of the gastro-duodenal contents into the esophagus [38, 39]. As a result of stasis of the refluxate material in the esophagus, patients can present with symptoms of heartburn and regurgitation. Damage to the mucosal lining of the esophagus ranges from mild inflammation to mucosal erosion and carcinoma [38, 39]. Numerous studies indicate that gastroesophageal reflux disease (GERD) is a common comorbidity in FM and that patients with FM are at a high risk of having gastroesophageal reflux disease (GERD). *Wang et al.* conducted a retrospective cohort analysis using a nationwide database and noted a bidirectional association between FM and GERD. The incidence of GERD in patients with FM was 12 per 1000 person-year in comparison to 7.6 per 1000 person-year in those with no FM, with an adjusted hazard ratio of 1.27. On the other hand, the incidence of FM in patients with GERD was 5.6 per 1000 person-year versus 3.96 per 1000.person-year in those with no GERD, with an adjusted hazard ratio of 1.44. The authors also noted a higher prevalence of peptic ulcer disease in FM patients in comparison to controls [40]. In a retrospective analysis on associated comorbidities in patients with FM, *Rivera et al.* reported the prevalence of GERD among other GI disorders such as IBS. Furthermore, GERD was significantly associated with worse treatment outcome in terms of pain and functionality. The study group consisted of 411 patients who were included in a cognitive behavioral treatment program in a tertiary care center [41]. *Pamuk et al.* investigated the GI symptoms in 152 women diagnosed with FM and found a higher prevalence of reflux, belching and bloating in comparison to controls and to another group diagnosed with rheumatoid arthritis. Moreover, FM patients had significantly higher scores for dyspepsia-related quality of life disturbances in comparison to the other two groups. The authors stressed the adverse effect of upper GI symptoms, particularly dyspepsia, on the quality of life of patients with FM [42]. In a systematic review on swallowing problems in adult FM patients, *Gilheany et al.* reported the prevalence of dysphagia and GERD in 51.9% and 25.9% of the cases, respectively. The authors stressed the adverse effects of swallowing disorders on quality of life of affected patients, particularly the increased risk of aspiration and the need for dietary change as a precautious measure [43]. *Savin et al.* conducted a retrospective cross-sectional study on the prevalence of GI disorders in a large cohort of patients with FM (n = 18,598) and noted a significant correlation between GERD and FM. The odds of having GERD in FM patients in comparison to controls was 2.62. Fibromyalgia patients were significantly more likely to have IBS, celiac disease, CD and UC with odd ratios of 4.61, 2.08, 1.85 and 1.82, respectively. The authors concluded that there was a positive correlation between benign GI disorders and FM [44].

The Impact of GERD in FM Patients on Voice

Many patients with GERD present with extraesophageal symptoms in the absence of heartburn and regurgitation [45, 46]. The most common are throat clearing, foreign body sensation, globus pharynges, intractable cough, and change in voice quality [47]. These symptoms occur mostly during the day and while the patient is in the upright position. The distinctive clinical presentation of patients with extra-esophageal symptoms of reflux and the normal upper endoscopy in the majority of these cases were suggestive of a new disease entity. Different terms have been used to describe it such as reflux laryngitis, extraesophageal reflux, supra-esophageal reflux and/or atypical reflux [48]. In 1991, *Koufman et al.* used the term laryngopharyngeal reflux (LPR) to denote a spectrum of throat symptoms in patients presenting to the otolaryngology practice with no classical symptoms of GERD. Laryngopharyngeal reflux is a common condition that affects 8–20% of the general population [49]. Many reports indicate that LPR is present in more than 50% of patients presenting with voice disorders and up to 75% of patients with refractory ENT symptoms [50–52].

There are no studies in the literature on the prevalence of LPR in FM. However, given the high prevalence of GERD in FM and the link between GERD and LPR, one can extrapolate that FM patients experience the extra-esophageal signs and symptoms of reflux disease. This extrapolation is based on the fact that LPR and GERD represent a spectrum of one disease despite the difference in the presenting symptoms and response to treatment [53–58]. *Groome et al.* conducted a study looking at the prevalence of LPR in 1383 patients proven to have GERD by upper gastrointestinal endoscopy and noted higher scores of Reflux symptom Index (RSI) in those with severe GERD in comparison to those with moderate, mild or inactive disease. For instance, the mean rating of hoarseness was 1.70 in patients with severe GERD versus 1.05 in those with inactive disease. Their findings strongly supported the hypothesis that LPR is a supra-esophageal manifestation of GERD despite the fact that LPR patients rarely experience the classical symptoms of GERD [57]. In an investigation on laryngeal signs of GERD, *Ylitalo et al.* noted a higher prevalence of pharyngeal acid reflux in patients with posterior laryngitis compared to those with a normal larynx (69% vs. 53%, respectively) [58]. In a study that included 169 patients diagnosed with reflux esophagitis, *Lai YC* reported the prevalence of LPR in 23.9% of the cases. There was a strong association between LPR and hiatal hernia among other factors such as age and hoarseness [59]. Other studies have also shown that LPR patients have diminished esophageal motility similar to what is observed in patients with GERD but to a lesser extent. This corroborates further the strong link between LPR and GERD [60–62].

In view of all the above, LPR may be an overlooked comorbidity that can contribute to the development of voice disorders in FM. The link between reflux disease, inflammatory and neoplastic diseases of the laryngopharyngeal complex is well documented in the literature [50, 52, 63–65]. *Wiener et al.* reported the presence of LPR using 24–h pH-metry in 78% of patients with chronic hoarseness, a figure that was corroborated by *Koufman* et al. and many others asserting the etiologic role of reflux in patients with dysphonia [52, 66–68]. *Wang et al.* evaluated the association between pepsin and vocal fold polyps using 24-h impedance-pH monitoring and immunohistochemical analysis of tissue samples taken from polyps. Results showed a significantly higher expression of pepsin expression in VFPs patients in comparison to controls (75% vs. 31.25%; P < .001). Moreover, there was a positive correlation between pepsin levels and outcome measures of 24 h impedance-pH monitoring in the upright position [67]. *Lu et al.* evaluated the etiologic role of LPR in vocal fold leukoplakia in 81 patients and noted the presence of acidic LPR and weakly acidic LPR in 35.8% and 43.2% of the patients, respectively [68].

In summary, GERD is a common comorbidity in FM. The retrograde movement of the gastroesophageal contents may exacerbate pain sensitivity and central sensitization. Affected patients suffer from an array of symptoms related to the laryngopharyngeal complex including hoarseness. Physicians should be alert about the increased risk of structural and functional voice disorders in FM patients with reflux disease.

References

1. Yunus M, Masi AT, Calabro JJ, Miller KA, Feigenbaum SL. Primary fibromyalgia (fibrositis): clinical study of 50 patients with matched normal controls. Semin Arthritis Rheum. 1981;11(1):151–71.
2. Triadafilopoulos G, Simms RW, Goldenberg DL. Bowel dysfunction in fibromyalgia syndrome. Dig Dis Sci. 1991;36(1):59–64.

3. Slim M, Calandre EP, Rico-Villademoros F. An insight into the gastrointestinal component of fibromyalgia: clinical manifestations and potential underlying mechanisms. Rheumatol Int. 2015;35(3):433–44.
4. Erdrich S, Hawrelak JA, Myers SP, Harnett JE. A systematic review of the association between fibromyalgia and functional gastrointestinal disorders. Ther Adv Gastroenterol. 2020;13:1756284820977402.
5. Clauw DJ. Fibromyalgia: a clinical review. JAMA. 2014;311(15):1547–55.
6. Malt EA, Ursin H. Mutilation anxiety differs among females with fibromyalgia and functional dyspepsia and population controls. J Psychosom Res. 2003;54(6):523–31.
7. Cho HS, Park JM, Lim CH, Cho YK, Lee IS, Kim SW, Choi MG, Chung IS, Chung YK. Anxiety, depression and quality of life in patients with irritable bowel syndrome. Gut Liver. 2011;5(1):29–36.
8. Barberio B, Zamani M, Black CJ, Savarino EV, Ford AC. Prevalence of symptoms of anxiety and depression in patients with inflammatory bowel disease: a systematic review and meta-analysis. Lancet Gastroenterol Hepatol. 2021;6(5):359–70.
9. Miwa H, Kondo T, Oshima T. Gastroesophageal reflux disease-related and functional heartburn: pathophysiology and treatment. Curr Opin Gastroenterol. 2016;32(4):344–52.
10. Konturek PC, Brzozowski T, Konturek SJ. Stress and the gut: pathophysiology, clinical consequences, diagnostic approach and treatment options. J Physiol Pharmacol. 2011;62(6):591–9.
11. Wallace DJ, Hallegua DS. Fibromyalgia: the gastrointestinal link. Curr Pain Headache Rep. 2004;8(5):364–8.
12. Huang CS, Farraye FA. Irritable bowel syndrome: managing this complex disorder. Womens Health Prim Care. 2003;6:247–56.
13. Staudacher HM, Black CJ, Teasdale SB, Mikocka-Walus A, Keefer L. Irritable bowel syndrome and mental health comorbidity—approach to multidisciplinary management. Nat Rev Gastroenterol Hepatol. 2023;20(9):582–96.
14. Cook IJ, van Eeden A, Collins SM. Patients with irritable bowel syndrome have greater pain tolerance than normal subjects. Gastroenterology. 1987;93(4):727–33.
15. Serra J, Azpiroz F, Malagelada JR. Impaired transit and tolerance of intestinal gas in the irritable bowel syndrome. Gut. 2001;48(1):14–9.
16. Lee HJ, Choi E, Nahm FS, Choi SS, Kim YH, Moon JY, Kim SH, Cho CW, Lee PB. Prevalence of fibromyalgia in fourteen Korean tertiary care university hospital pain clinics. J Pain Res. 2018;11:2417–23.
17. Fond G, Loundou A, Hamdani N, Boukouaci W, Dargel A, Oliveira J, Roger M, Tamouza R, Leboyer M, Boyer L. Anxiety and depression comorbidities in irritable bowel syndrome (IBS): a systematic review and meta-analysis. Eur Arch Psychiatry Clin Neurosci. 2014;264(8):651–60.
18. Diao Z, Xu W, Guo D, Zhang J, Zhang R, Liu F, Hu Y, Ma Y. Causal association between psycho-psychological factors, such as stress, anxiety, depression, and irritable bowel syndrome: Mendelian randomization. Medicine (Baltimore). 2023;102(34):e34802.
19. Enin K, Parikh A, Kallogjeri D, Naunheim MR, Huston MN. Correlation between a diagnosis of anxiety or depression and initial VHI-10 scores in benign dysphonia. Otolaryngol Head Neck Surg. 2022;167(4):725–30.
20. Maksimovic JM, Vukasinovic MM, Vlajinac HD, Jotic AD, Milovanovic MS, Ivanov SY, Maksimovic MZ, Milovanovic JP. Anxiety and depression in patients with vocal fold nodules, edema and polyps. Eur Arch Otorrinolaringol. 2020;277(9):2493–500.
21. Montgomery J, Hendry J, Wilson JA, Deary IJ, MacKenzie K. Pragmatic detection of anxiety and depression in a prospective cohort of voice outpatient clinic attenders. Clin Otolaryngol. 2016;41(1):2–7.
22. Sheth T, Pitchumoni CS, Das KM. Musculoskeletal manifestations in inflammatory bowel disease: a revisit in search of immunopathophysiological mechanisms. J Clin Gastroenterol. 2014;48(4):308–17.
23. Saeid Seyedian S, Nokhostin F, et al. A review of the diagnosis, prevention, and treatment methods of inflammatory bowel disease. J Med Life. 2019;12:113–22.

24. Guan Q. A comprehensive review and update on the pathogenesis of inflammatory bowel disease. J Immunol Res. 2019;2019:7247238.
25. Chen JH, Chen HJ, Kao CH, Tseng CH, Tsai CH. Is fibromyalgia risk higher among male and young inflammatory bowel disease patients? Evidence from a Taiwan cohort of one million. Pain Physician. 2018;21(3):E257–64.
26. Buskila D, Odes LR, Neumann L, Odes HS. Fibromyalgia in inflammatory bowel disease. J Rheumatol. 1999;26(5):1167–71.
27. Greenbaum H, Weil C, Chodick G, Shalev V, Eisenberg VH. Evidence for an association between endometriosis, fibromyalgia, and autoimmune diseases. Am J Reprod Immunol. 2019;81(4):e13095.
28. Rickli H, Fretz C, Hoffman M, Walser A, Knoblauch A. Severe inflammatory upper airway stenosis in ulcerative colitis. Eur Respir J. 1994;7(10):1899–902.
29. Hasegawa N, Ishimoto S, Takazoe M, Tsunoda K, Fujimaki Y, Shiraishi A, Kinoshita M, Okada K. Recurrent hoarseness due to inflammatory vocal fold lesions in a patient with Crohn's disease. Ann Otol Rhinol Laryngol. 2009;118(7):532–5.
30. Loos E, Lemkens P, Poorten VV, Humblet E, Laureyns G. Laryngeal manifestations of inflammatory bowel disease. J Voice. 2019;33(1):1–6.
31. Tahir E, Ustaoğlu M, Yaşar ÖC. Evaluation of voice in inflammatory bowel diseases. Folia Phoniatr Logop. 2024;76(5):458–66.
32. Bain WM, Harrington JW, Thomas LE, Schaefer SD. Head and neck manifestations of gastroesophageal reflux. Laryngoscope. 1983;93(2):175–9.
33. Richter JE, Rubenstein JH. Presentation and epidemiology of gastroesophageal reflux disease. Gastroenterology. 2018;154(2):267–76.
34. Karkos PD, Thomas L, Temple RH, Issing WJ. Awareness of general practitioners towards treatment of laryngopharyngeal reflux: a British survey. Otolaryngol Head Neck Surg. 2005;133(4):505–8.
35. El-Serag HB, Sweet S, Winchester CC, Dent J. Update on the epidemiology of gastro-oesophageal reflux disease: a systematic review. Gut. 2014;63(6):871–80.
36. Locke G, Talley N, Fett S, Zinsmeister A, Melton L. Prevalence and clinical spectrum of gastroesophageal reflux: a population-based study in Olmsted County, Minnesota. Gastroenterology. 1997;112(5):1448–56.
37. Altman KW, Stephens RM, Lyttle CS, Weiss KB. Changing impact of gastroesophageal reflux in medical and otolaryngology practice. Laryngoscope. 2005;115(7):1145–53.
38. Olson NR. Effects of stomach acid on the larynx. Proc Am Laryngol Assoc. 1983;104(104):108–12.
39. Ohman L, Olofsson J, Tibbling L, Ericsson G. Esophageal dysfunction in patients with contact ulcer of the larynx. Ann Otol Rhinol Laryngol. 1983;92(3 Pt 1):228–30.
40. Wang JC, Sung FC, Men M, Wang KA, Lin CL, Kao CH. Bidirectional association between fibromyalgia and gastroesophageal reflux disease: two population-based retrospective cohort analysis. Pain. 2017;158(10):1971–8.
41. Rivera FA, Munipalli B, Allman ME, Hodge DO, Wieczorek MA, Wang B, Abril A, Perlman A, Knight D, Bruce B. A retrospective analysis of the prevalence and impact of associated comorbidities on fibromyalgia outcomes in a tertiary care center. Front Med (Lausanne). 2024;10:1301944.
42. Pamuk ON, Umit H, Harmandar O. Increased frequency of gastrointestinal symptoms in patients with fibromyalgia and associated factors: a comparative study. J Rheumatol. 2009;36(8):1720–4.
43. Gilheaney Ó, Chadwick A. The prevalence and nature of eating and swallowing problems in adults with fibromyalgia: a systematic review. Dysphagia. 2024;39(1):92–108.
44. Savin E, Tsur AM, Watad A, Gendelman O, Kopylov U, Cohen AD, Amital H. Association of fibromyalgia with cancerous and non-cancerous gastrointestinal comorbidities: a cross-sectional study. Clin Exp Rheumatol. 2023;41(6):1248–53.
45. Feder RJ, Michell MJ. Hyperfunctional, hyperacidic, and intubation granulomas. Arch Otolaryngol. 1984;110(9):582–4.

46. Belmont JR, Grundfast K. Congenital laryngeal stridor (laryngomalacia): etiologic factors and associated disorders. Ann Otol Rhinol Laryngol. 1984;93(5):430–7.
47. Book DT, Rhee JS, Toohill RJ, Smith TL. Perspectives in laryngopharyngeal reflux: an international survey. Laryngoscope. 2002;112(8):1399–406.
48. Pontes P, Tiago R. Diagnosis and management of laryngopharyngeal reflux disease. Curr Opin Otolaryngol Head Neck Surg. 2006;14(3):138–42.
49. Rees LE, Pazmany L, Gutowska-Owsiak D, Inman CF, Phillips A, Stokes CR, Johnston N, Koufman JA, Postma G, Bailey M, Birchall MA. The mucosal immune response to laryngopharyngeal reflux. Am J Respir Crit Care Med. 2008;177(11):1187–93.
50. Ward PH, Zwitman D, Hanson D, Berci G. Contact ulcers and granulomas of the larynx: new insights into their etiology as a basis for more rational treatment. Otolaryngol Head Neck Surg (1979). 1980;88(3):262–9.
51. Sataloff RT, Spiegel JR, Hawkshaw MJ. Strobovideolaryngoscopy: results and clinical value. Ann Otol Rhinol Laryngol. 1991;100(9 Pt 1):725–7.
52. Koufman JA, Wiener GJ, Wu WC, Castell DO. Reflux laryngitis and its sequelae: the diagnostic role of ambulatory 24-hour pH monitoring. J Voice. 1988;2(1):78–89.
53. Halstead LA. Role of gastroesophageal reflux in pediatric upper airway disorders. Otolaryngol Head Neck Surg. 1999;120(2):208–14.
54. Al-Sabbagh G, Wo JM. Supraesophageal manifestations of gastroesophageal reflux disease. Semin Gastrointest Dis. 1999;10(3):113–9.
55. Hanson DG, Jiang JJ. Diagnosis and management of chronic laryngitis associated with reflux. Am J Med. 2000;108(Suppl 4a):112S–9S.
56. GrøntvedAM, West F. PH monitoring in patients with benign voice disorders. Acta Otolaryngol Suppl. 2000;543:229–31.
57. Groome M, Cotton JP, Borland M, McLeod S, Johnston DA, Dillon JF. Prevalence of laryngopharyngeal reflux in a population with gastroesophageal reflux. Laryngoscope. 2007;117(8):1424–8.
58. Ylitalo RH, Lindestad P-A, Ramel S. Symptoms, laryngeal findings and 24-hour 2-site pH monitoring in patients with suspected gastroesophago-pharyngeal reflux. Gastroenterology. 2001;120(5):A426.
59. Lai Y-C, Wang P, Lin J. Laryngopharyngeal reflux in patients with reflux esophagitis. World J Gastroenterol. 2008;14(28):4523.
60. Helm JF, Dodds WJ, Hogan WJ, Soergel KH, Egide MS, Wood CM. Acid neutralizing capacity of human saliva. Gastroenterology. 1982;83(1 Pt 1):69–74.
61. Knight RE, Wells JR, Parrish RS. Esophageal dysmotility as an important Co-factor in extraesophageal manifestations of gastroesophageal reflux. Laryngoscope. 2000;110(9):1462–6.
62. Sataloff RT, Castell DO, Kaltz PO, Sataloff DM. Reflux laryngitis and related disorders. 3rd ed. San Diego: Plural Publishing; 2006.
63. Ross JA, Noordzji JP, Woo P. Voice disorders in patients with suspected laryngo-pharyngeal reflux disease. J Voice. 1998;12(1):84–8.
64. Rothstein SG. Reflux and vocal disorders in singers with bulimia. J Voice. 1998;12(1):89–90.
65. Kuhn J, Toohill RJ, Ulualp SO, Kulpa J, Hofmann C, Arndorfer R, Shaker R. Pharyngeal acid reflux events in patients with vocal cord nodules. Laryngoscope. 1998;108(8 Pt 1):1146–9.
66. Toohill RJ, Ulualp SO, Shaker R. Evaluation of gastroesophageal reflux in patients with laryngotracheal stenosis. Ann Otol Rhinol Laryngol. 1998;107(12):1010–4.
67. Wang L, Tan JJ, Wu T, Zhang R, Wu JN, Zeng FF, Liu YL, Han XY, Li YF, Li XP. Association between laryngeal pepsin levels and the presence of vocal fold polyps. Otolaryngol Head Neck Surg. 2017;156(1):144–51.
68. Lu G, Ding X, Xu W. Association between laryngopharyngeal reflux and vocal fold leukoplakia. ORL J Otorhinolaryngol Relat Spec. 2021;83(3):159–66.

8 Rheumatologic Diseases in Fibromyalgia and Impact on Voice

Abdul-latif Hamdan, Robert Thayer Sataloff, and Mary J. Hawkshaw

Fibromyalgia (FM) is a disorder characterized by widespread musculoskeletal pain associated with diffuse body aches and point tenderness. Affected patients suffer from a large number of comorbidities that worsen their quality of life and often mask the diagnosis. Many of these comorbidities are related to central nervous system dysregulation such as irritable bowel syndrome and painful bladder syndrome, and many are related to autoimmune and peripheral inflammatory disorders [1]. Among those are rheumatoid arthritis (RA), Systemic lupus erythematosus (SLE), Sjogren Syndrome (SS), ankylosis spondylosis (AS) and osteoarthritis (OA). Physicians should be familiar with the link between rheumatologic diseases and FM, and on their potential adverse effect on voice.

The Link Between RA and FM

Rheumatoid arthritis is chronic inflammatory disorder that affects almost 1% of the world population with women being affected more than men [2]. The disease targets primarily the articular and extra-articular surfaces of diarthrodial joints leading to tissue destruction and functional disability [3, 4]. Numerous studies have been published on the coexistence of FM and RA, showing that a large percentage of patients with FM experience symptoms of RA and vice-versa [5–8]. In a study that included 202 patients with RA, *Gao et al.* reported FM in 20.8% of the cases. The authors highlighted the need to consider FM as a comorbidity in RA patients refractory to treatment [5]. In a review on the clinical course of patients with inflammatory arthritis including RA, *Zhao et al.* reported pooled prevalence of FM between 18% and 24% of the cases. The authors advocated for early recognition of FM patients with rheumatologic disorders [6]. The coexistence of FM and RA worsens the clinical picture and functional ability of affected subjects. In a retrospective analysis of FM patients undergoing cognitive behavioral therapy, *Rivera et al.* noted RA as one of

A.-l. Hamdan et al., *Voice Disorders in Fibromyalgia*, https://doi.org/10.1007/978-3-031-97751-0_8

many comorbidities that affected treatment adversely. The study included 411 participants who were managed in a tertiary referral center [7]. In a review on centralized pain in FM patients, *Minhas et al.* found that those with concomitant RA had worse disease activity score than those without RA. The authors ascribed that difference to central processing of the nociplastic pain experienced by diseased subjects [8]. *Durmaz et al.* conducted a cross-sectional study comparing RA disease activity in RA patients with and without FM and found higher median values of Disease Activity Scores-28 (DAS28) in those with concomitant FM. There was also a significant difference in the median values of tender joint count and patient global assessment between those with and without FM [9]. In a study by *Gao et al,* the coexistence of FM in RA patients increased significantly the tender joint score, disease activity score, as well as the health assessment questionnaire score. The authors opined about the need to rule out FM in RA patients who do not achieve remission despite therapy [5].

Impact of RA on Voice in FM Patients

There are no reports in the literature on voice disorders in FM patients with RA. However, there are many on the impact of RA on voice. As the larynx is a musculoskeletal organ with diarthrodial joints, it is subject to the manifestation of rheumatologic disorders including RA. Histologic studies have shown involvement of different laryngeal structures in up to 88% of patients with RA [5–12]. Affected patients may complain of voice fatigue, breathiness, loss of volume, disturbance in pitch, dysphagia, odynophagia, and aspiration. Using a phone survey, *Roy et al.* reported throat-related complaints in 35% of affected patients with the most significant ones being throat discomfort and dryness [13–15]. Voice and swallowing symptoms in the early stage of the disease are attributed to inflammation of the posterior laryngeal and pharyngeal mucosa. *Kirgezen et al.* investigated the phonatory disorders of patients with RA and noted posterior commissure hypertrophy and hyperemia/edema in 25.3% and 22.3% of cases, respectively. The prevalence of abnormal laryngeal findings increased with disease severity [16]. Patients with long-standing RA also can present with shortness of breath, stridor and respiratory distress secondary to impaired mobility of the vocal folds and narrowing of the glottic aperture [17–20]. *Jurik et al.* reported a female patient with RA who presented with stridor secondary to fixation of both vocal folds in the midline. Radiologic evaluation revealed erosion of the cricoarytenoid joint (CAJ) structures suggestive of chronic arthritis. The patient was treated successfully with steroids [21]. *Meng et al.* reviewed the medical records and clinical data of 31 patients with autoimmune diseases including 17 cases of RA, and found that vocal fold fixation was one of the most common laryngeal findings (38.7%). Systemic treatment improved the voice symptoms in almost 45% of the study group [22]. *Leicht et al.* highlighted the need to recognize this condition during the work-up of patients presenting with stridor in order to avoid delay in diagnosis and therapy, as well as compromised treatment outcomes [23].

Other rare laryngeal findings in RA include rheumatoid nodules. Rheumatoid nodules are submucosal masses that can be found in the CAJ, on the vocal folds or in the peri-arytenoid area [24]. Histologic examination invariably shows necrotic, eosinophilic staining with an outer rim of fibrosis [25]. In symptomatic patients, micro-laryngeal surgery is the treatment of choice. Bamboo nodes are another rare laryngeal finding in RA. Bamboo nodes are yellowish, transverse submucosal masses on the vocal folds in patients with autoimmune disease. They were described first by *Hosako et al.* in 1993 as a cause of dysphonia in a 39-year-old-female patient diagnosed with undifferentiated connective tissue disease [26]. The lesion consists histologically of an ill-defined inflammatory mass with central necrosis surrounded by macrophages [27]. Voice therapy and the use of immunosuppressant medication usually were beneficial in the management of these lesions. Alternative therapy is steroid injection and surgery.

The Link Between SS and FM

Sjogren syndrome (SS) is a chronic autoimmune disorder with a diverse clinical presentation. It is labelled as primary when it occurs in isolation and secondary when it arises in the context of another autoimmune disease. Lymphocytic infiltration of various exocrine organs is the hallmark of this syndrome that often is associated with an increased risk for non-Hodgkin B cell lymphoma. Oral and ocular dryness are the most common complaints, often associated with dysgeusia and infections of the oral cavity [28]. Systemic complaints such as body fatigue and aches also may arise as a result of extra-glandular disease involvement. Diagnosis of SS is based on the clinical presentation and serologic markers that show the presence of antinuclear auto-antibodies (anti-Ro/SSA and anti-La/SSB, ANA and RF) [28]. Treatment focuses on symptom relief and managing the systemic manifestations. The sicca symptoms usually are managed by artificial tears and saliva substitutes in addition to lifestyle changes that include good hydration and oral hygiene. Pilocarpine is recommended in refractory cases. In patients with severe systemic complaints, immunosuppressants and targeted biologic therapies are advocated [29].

The link between SS and Fibromyalgia FM is a subject of growing interest because of the significant overlap in the clinical presentation of the disease entities. While diffuse pain and body fatigue are cardinal symptoms of FM, they are also common complaints in patients with SS. Similarly, diagnostic features of SS such as a dryness in the mouth and eyes are reported frequently in FM patients [30]. There are numerous studies on the co-existence of FM and SS. In 2019, *Applbaum et al.* tested 151 FM patients who complained of sicca symptoms and noted SS in 32%. The authors used several biomarkers for the diagnosis of SS including SS-autoantibodies, antinuclear antibodies (ANA), and rheumatoid factor (RF) [28]. In 2021, *Gau et al.* investigated the risk of SS in a Nationwide population-based cohort that included 74,853 FM patients and reported an adjusted hazard ratio (aHR) of 2.00

(95% CI). The aHR increased to 3.07 (95% CI) in those between the age of 20 and 49 years. The authors discussed the high risk of SS in FM patients and the need to consider and manage this syndrome in the management of affected patients [31]. Numerous studies also showed a high prevalence of FM in patients with SS. In 2008, *D. Elia et al.* investigated the prevalence of fatigue in 48 women with SS using the Multidimensional Fatigue Inventory (MFI-20) [32] and found significantly higher scores in comparison to controls in all subscales of the questionnaire. The scores of SS patients were comparable to those of FM patients [33]. In 2016, *Choi et al.* examined 100 patients with primary SS and noted that 31% had clinical features of FM based on the American College of Rheumatology (ACR) 2010 criteria [34]. Moreover, there was a significant correlation between the European Alliance of Associations for Rheumatology (EULAR) Sjogren Syndrome Patient Reported Index and the Widespread Pain Index (WPI) and the symptom severity scale (SSS). The risk of FM increased in patients with SS and depression, and in patients with a low serum 25-hydroxy vitamin D3 level [35]. In 2021, *Dubost et al.* investigated the prevalence of FM in 134 patients with SS using different diagnostic criteria and noted a prevalence rate between 18% and 29% [36]. Eighteen percent of the study group had FM using the ACR 2016 [37] in comparison to 29% using the Fibromyalgia Rapid Screening Tool (FiRST) [38].

Impact of SS on Voice in FM Patients

There are no published studies on voice disorders in FM patients with SS. However, there are numerous reports on SS and voice disorders and on the adverse effect of oral dryness (xerostomia) on voice production [39]. *Pierce et al.* investigated the prevalence of voice disorders in 101 patients with SS using validated questionnaires and showed that more than half (59.4%) had vocal complaints that progressed over time and became chronic. The authors stressed the high frequency of voice-related symptoms in SS patients and the need to address these symptoms in the treatment of SS [40]. *Salturk et al.* evaluated the voices of ten patients with SS and noted a significantly higher VHI-10 score in comparison to controls. Laryngeal videostroboscopic examination showed differences in glottic closure and smoothness of the vocal folds between the two groups [41]. *Heller et al.* reported a significant difference in amplitude perturbation quotient, shimmer and average fundamental frequency in patients with SS compared to normative values. The differences in acoustic measures were substantiated by an elevated Cepstral Spectral Index of Dysphonia for connected speech and sustained vowels. Patients also were noted to have mild-to-moderate dysphonia using the Visual Analog Scale (VAS). Their findings were associated with dryness of the laryngeal mucosa as seen on videolaryngostroboscopic examination [42].

The high prevalence of voice disorders in SS can be ascribed to laryngeal desiccation associated with hyposalivation. Numerous studies indicate that dryness of the vocal folds associated and oral dryness increase the prevalence of vocal fatigue and phonatory effort [43–45]. In a study on the effect of mouth breathing on voice,

Sivasankar et al. reported an increase in phonatory threshold pressure at low and high humidity. The phonatory threshold pressure is the pressure needed to set the vocal folds into vibration and is the correlate of phonatory effort [46]. *Hira et al.* investigated the impact of dry mouth on voice by measuring the volume of saliva in a cohort of 232 patients with COPD or asthma. The results showed an inverse relation between salivation and degree of self-perceived hoarseness. Hyposalivation was found to be a significant predictor of hoarseness with an accuracy of 0.69, 95% CI. The prediction accuracy increased in patients treated with fluticasone [47]. *Lee et al.* investigated the voice characteristics of 1197 patients with adeno-tonsillar disease admitted for surgery and noted that 91 had dysphonia based on auditory perceptual ratings. The authors ascribed the change in voice quality to mouth breathing and poor vocal hygiene [48]. The adverse effect of dehydration on voice also has been investigated in the context of religious rituals such as fasting. Studies have shown that abstention from water intake for more than 12 h resulted in voice fatigue and increase in phonatory effort [49, 50]. Based on these studies, one can extrapolate that FM patients with co-existent SS are at higher risk of having voice disorders as a result of oral and laryngeal dryness. The increase in phonatory effort reported by affected patients is a risk factor for functional and structural voice disorders. Future studies on the prevalence and causes of dysphonia in patients with FM and SS are warranted.

Another cause of hoarseness in SS patients is cricoarytenoid joint arthritis with or without fixation of the vocal fold. *Seve et al.* reported a 50-year-old-female patient with history of polyarthralgia who presented with dysphonia and had asymmetry of the arytenoid cartilages with mucosal edema on laryngeal examination suggestive of cricoarytenoid arthritis. The patient was diagnosed with SS and was started on prednisolone. On follow up, she had marked improvement in her symptoms and in her laryngeal findings [51]. Other rare causes of hoarseness in SS include vocal fold masses secondary to lymphocytic infiltration [52], vocal fold nodules [53], and bamboo nodes [54]. *Todic et al.* reviewed the medical records of ten patients with vocal fold bamboo nodes and noted the diagnosis of SS in one of them. The authors highlighted that those autoimmune diseases often are overlooked in the work up of patients with dysphonia [54]. *Hanai et al.* reported a 27-year-old-women who presented with hoarseness secondary to a vocal fold bamboo node. The patient tested positive for anti-SS-A and anti-SS-B antibodies and underwent microlaryngeal resection of her vocal fold lesion which revealed hyaline degeneration and submucosal fibrosis [55].

The Link Between SLE and FM

Systemic Lupus erythematosus (SLE) is a systemic autoimmune disease that affects various organs in the body. As a result of progressive tissue damage, patients present with many systemic complaints and cognitive dysfunction in various domains. The symptoms are heterogenous and not always confined to one organ. Among those reported commonly are myalgia, diffuse body pain and arthralgia. The musculoskeletal symptoms and the diffuse widespread pain often coincide with symptoms of FM making the diagnosis of SLE very difficult [56]. In a systematic review and meta-analysis on the risk of FM in patients with SLE, *Mistry et al.* reported an odds ratio of 3.7 (95%CI). The pooled prevalence of FM was 15.8% [57]. In another review on SLE, *Staud R et al.* found that 47% of SLE patients fulfilled the diagnostic criteria of FM. However, the co-existence of FM was not predictive of tissue damage, nor did it worsen the prognosis [58]. *Middleton et al.* investigated the prevalence of FM in 102 patients with SLE and noted that 45% met the diagnostic criteria for FM or had symptoms suggestive of FM. Despite the high prevalence of FM as a secondary diagnosis in SLE patients, it is important to note the lack of a correlation between disease activity of SLE and FM [59]. In a retrospective cohort that included 72 SLE patients who underwent musculoskeletal ultrasound for joint pain, *Song et al.* found that 43.1% of their study population had a pre-existing diagnosis of FM [60]. *Kotter et al.* reported a higher prevalence of SLE in patients with Fibromyalgia in comparison to the general population (0.8% vs. 0.05%, respectively) while investigating the prevalence of autoimmune diseases in patients with FM [61].

Impact of SLE on Voice in FM Patients

No studies have been published on voice characteristics of FM patients with SLE. However, there are a few studies and case reports on the prevalence of voice disorders in SLE patients. In 2001, *Murano et al.* reported two cases of vocal fold bamboo nodes, one of whom was diagnosed with SLE. The authors highlighted that hoarseness and the presence of a whitish submucosal vocal fold lesion might be the presenting symptom and sign of SLE and that they should prompt physicians to investigate for autoimmune diseases [62]. In 2008, *Lee et al.* reported a 41-year-old-female patient who was known to have SLE who presented with hoarseness and other systemic complaints. The patient was diagnosed with unilateral vocal fold palsy, and laryngeal electromyography (LEMG) showed signs of denervation and reinnervation. The authors highlighted the laryngeal manifestation of SLE and the role of LEMG in diagnosing neuromuscular dysfunction in affected patients [63]. *In 2013, Leszczynnski and Pawlak-Bus* reported a 38-year-old-female patient with SLE who presented with a history of hoarseness. On laryngeal examination, she had bilateral vocal fold paralysis. The patient had high levels of antinuclear antibodies suggestive of an autoimmune disease, among other comorbidities [64]. In 2017, *De Macedo et al.* investigated the prevalence of voice disorders in a cohort of patients diagnosed with SLE and reported a voice deficit in 29 out of the 36 participants. The most common symptoms were voice fatigue and hoarseness. These self-reported complaints correlated with an increase in auditory perceptual ratings, an increase in the perturbation parameters, and a decrease in voice intensity. The authors stressed the need to address voice complaints in SLE patients in order to improve the overall quality of life of affected patients [65]. In 2018, *Todic et al.* conducted a retrospective review of ten patients diagnosed with Bamboo nodes and found that three of those had SLE. The authors noted that SLE should be included in the work-up of patients with Bamboo nodes [54].

The Link Between Ankylosing Spondylitis and FM

Ankylosing Spondylitis (AS) is a form of arthritis that involves primarily the axial skeleton and sacroiliac joints. The disease affects one in a 200 people worldwide leading to functional disability and decrease in quality of life [66]. The pathogenesis of AS remains unknown. A genetic background has been suggested in view of the high prevalence of genetic polymorphisms in affected patients, and the most significant association is with HLA B 27. In addition to the genome-wide association, immune and inflammatory pathways have been implicated such as the interleukin-17/IL-23 pathways [67, 68]. Changes in microbiota and stress also have been suggested as playing a role in the pathogenesis of this disease [66]. A cardinal symptom of AS is progressive chronic back pain. Affected patients usually are treated initially with non-steroidal anti-inflammatory medications. In more advanced cases, the use of tumor necrosis inhibitor therapy has been advocated [66].

The link between AS and FM has been reported by many authors. In 2007, Aloush *et al.* assessed the prevalence of FM in 18 women with AS and found that half of them were affected. In comparison to men with AS, women with AS and FM had higher number of tender points and worse disease activity. There was also a correlation between the Bath AS disease activity and the number of tender points [69]. The Batch Ankylosing Spondylitis Functional Index (BASFI) is an index used to assess physical function in patients with AS. It uses self-reported response to ten questions related to activities of daily living scored from 0 (normal) to 10 (maximal impairment) [70]. In 2010, in a cross-sectional study which included 462 patients with AS, *Almodovar et al.* reported the prevalence of FM in 10. 8% of female patients. This risk of FM increased when the ratio of Bath AS disease activity index to Bath AS radiology index exceeded 1.5, or when the ratio of Bath AS functional index to Bath AS radiology index exceeded 1.08 [71]. In 2021, *Baraka et al.* investigated the co-existence of FM in patients with AS and noted a prevalence of 22.9%. Patients with AS and FM had a delay in diagnosis of AS, and more morning stiffness in comparison to AS patients without FM [71]. The authors concluded that AS patients with co-existing FM had worse quality of life and impaired function which warrants early screening [72]. In 2021, *Gau et al.* investigated the risk of FM in patients with AS and reported an adjusted hazard ratio of 1.32 (95% CI). The incidence rate per 1000 person-months was higher in AS patients compared to non-AS subjects (0.52 vs. 0.39, respectively). The authors used the National Taiwan Insurance Research Database which included 5.696 patients newly diagnosed with AS [73].

Impact of AS on Voice in FM Patients

There are no studies in the literature on voice disorders in FM patients with AS but there are reports on voice disorders in patients with AS who do not have FM. *Ahmed et al.* evaluated the voice of 32 patients with AS and found significantly lower values for maximum phonation time, fundamental frequency, jitter and shimmer in comparison to healthy controls. Moreover, patients with AS had higher eating assessment scores and penetration-aspiration scores using flexible endoscopic evaluation of swallowing. The authors highlighted the adverse effects of voice and swallowing disorders on quality of life of patients with AS. They also stressed the need for close observation to avoid aspiration [74]. Another rare cause of dysphonia in AS is cricoarytenoid arthritis with impaired mobility of the vocal fold. This laryngeal manifestation is relatively rare and occurs mostly in patients with a long history of AS. *Bienenstock and Lanyl* reported a 50-year-old woman, with known AS who presented with hoarseness and sore throat. The patient had fixation of the left vocal fold on laryngeal examination. She was treated successfully with steroids. However, the impaired mobility of the vocal fold recurred following cessation of therapy [75]. *Miller et al.* reported another case of AS who presented with dysphonia, dyspnea and stridor secondary to bilateral vocal fold fixation due to cricoarytenoid joint arthritis. The patient was treated with bilateral methylprednisolone acetate injection (40 mg/mL) of 0.5 ml into each cricoarytenoid joint [76]. Another rare laryngeal finding in AS is laryngocele. *Erdogmus et al.* were the first to report a case of laryngocele in a patient with AS. The authors attributed the development of the laryngocele to the increase in intralaryngeal pressure associated with the increase in intra-abdominal pressure due the Valsalva maneuver [77].

The Link Between OA and FM

Osteoarthritis (OA) is a chronic pain disorder that affects millions of people worldwide. Stress, psychological disturbances and genetic predisposition increase the risk for this disorder. The pathophysiology is complex. Central sensitization, alteration in pain processing and abnormal control of the descending pathways are some of the mechanisms suggested to explain the poor control of pain. Abnormal levels of interleukin-6, IL-10 and IL-1beta have been reported in affected patients [78, 79]. The link between OA and FM has been investigated by many authors. In a study on the frequency of FM in patients with knee OA, *Mahgoub et al.* reported a prevalence of 35.5%. Patients with OA and FM had poorer sleep quality and worse pain than those with OA and no FM. The authors stressed the adverse effects of FM on quality of life of patients with OA. Similarly, OA has been reported as a common comorbidity in patients with FM [80]. *Bernatsky et al.* investigated comorbidities in 180 women with FM and reported OA in 40% of the cases. Osteoarthritis was noted as one of the most common medical comorbidites in FM followed by irritable bowel syndrome. The presence of comorbidities in 90% of FM patients resulted in a significant increase in the number of medical visits [81]. *Haviland et al.* reviewed the comorbidities in hospitalized FM patients and reported co-existence of OA in 25–67% of cases. The data were extracted from the Nationwide inpatient sample (Nis) which included community and clinical facilities [82].

Impact of OA on Voice in Patients with FM

There are no studies published on the impact of OA on voice in FM patients, but there are a few on OA and voice. Given the similarity of the cricoarytenoid joint to other diarthrodial joints in the body, the reported cases are mostly on vocal fold fixation. In 1999. *Paulsen and Tillmann* examined 68 cricoarytenoid joints in cadaver of subjects above the age of 40 years and noted degenerative changes suggestive of OA in 50% of the cases. Histologic findings included loss of proteoglycans and fibrillated articular cartilage with alteration in the distribution of lectins. These subjects were from the general population, and medical history of conditions such as FM was not reported; but the specimens were taken from subjects who reportedly did not have" diseases which might involve or affect laryngeal function" (83, p. 505). The authors highlighted the adverse effect of these changes on vocal fold mobility [83]. In 2012, *Virk et al.* reported an elderly man who presented with a change in voice quality due to vocal fold fixation. The authors attributed immobility of the vocal fold to a large cervical osteophyte related to the long-standing history of osteoarthritis. The authors stressed the need to consider autoimmune diseases in the work-up of patients with an immobile vocal fold. The patient was treated conservatively with voice therapy and no surgical intervention was needed [84].

In summary, rheumatologic disorders are very common in FM with marked overlap in their clinical presentation. Systemic complaints such as body aches, fatigue, and early exhaustion may mask the diagnosis and delay treatment. The use of specific serologic biomarkers can assist in differentiating between the different disease entities. Patients with coexisting FM and rheumatologic disorders appear to be at a higher risk for developing voice disorders. Affected patients can present with hoarseness, dysphagia, odynophagia, aspiration and stridor. Common findings on laryngeal examination include edema and redness of the posterior larynx, vocal fold masses such as bamboo nodes, and unilateral or bilateral vocal fold immobility secondary to cricoarytenoid joint arthritis. Laryngeal examination of FM patients with dysphonia is essential to rule out structural and neurologic voice disorders. Treatment of the underlying rheumatologic disease may alleviate the voice symptoms. Laryngeal steroid injection in patients with vocal fold bamboo nodes and or cricoarytenoid joint arthritis is advocated in selected cases.

References

1. Lichtenstein A, Tiosano S, Amital H. The complexities of fibromyalgia and its comorbidities. Curr Opin Rheumatol. 2018;30(1):94–100.
2. Venetsanopoulou AI, Alamanos Y, Voulgari PV, Drosos AA. Epidemiology of rheumatoid arthritis: genetic and environmental influences. Expert Rev Clin Immunol. 2022;18(9):923–31.
3. Geterud Å. Rheumatoid arthritis in the larynx. Scand J Rheumatol. 1991;20(3):215.

4. Bienenstock H, Ehrlich GE, Freyberg RH. Rheumatoid arthritis of the cricoarytenoid joint: a clinicopathologic study. Arth Rheum. 1963;6(1):48–63.
5. Gao C, Zhong H, Chen L, Wang L, Yao H, Huang X, Jia Y, Li C, Liu T. Clinical and psychological assessment of patients with rheumatoid arthritis and fibromyalgia: a real-world study. Clin Rheumatol. 2022;41(4):1235–40.
6. Zhao SS, Duffield SJ, Goodson NJ. The prevalence and impact of comorbid fibromyalgia in inflammatory arthritis. Best Pract Res Clin Rheumatol. 2019;33(3):101423.
7. Rivera FA, Munipalli B, Allman ME, Hodge DO, Wieczorek MA, Wang B, Abril A, Perlman A, Knight D, Bruce B. A retrospective analysis of the prevalence and impact of associated comorbidities on fibromyalgia outcomes in a tertiary care center. Front Med (Lausanne). 2024;10:1301944.
8. Minhas D, Murphy A, Clauw DJ. Fibromyalgia and centralized pain in the rheumatoid arthritis patient. Curr Opin Rheumatol. 2023;35(3):170–4.
9. Durmaz Y, Ilhanli I. Rheumatoid arthritis activity scores in patients with and without fibromyalgia syndrome. Ann Saudi Med. 2021;41(4):246–52.
10. Amernik K. Glottis morphology and perceptive—acoustic characteristics of voice and speech in patients with rheumatoid arthritis [in Polish]. Ann Acad Med Stetin. 2007;53(3):55–65.
11. Wojnowski W, Karlik M, Wiskirska–Woznica B, Walczak M. Voice disorders in rheumatoid arthritis [in Polish]. Otolaryngol Pol. 2005;59(4):603–6.
12. Voulgari PV, Papazisi D, Bai M, Zagorianakou P, Assimakopoulos D, Drosos AA. Laryngeal involvement in rheumatoid arthritis. Rheumatol Int. 2005;25(5):321–5.
13. Roy N, Tanner K, Merrill RM, Wright C, Miller KL, Kendall KA. Descriptive epidemiology of voice disorders in rheumatoid arthritis: prevalence, risk factors, and quality of life burden. J Voice. 2016;30(1):74–87.
14. Masilamani K, Gandhi A. Cricoarytenoid arthritis presenting as croup. J Royal Soc Med. 2009;102(11):491–2.
15. Castro MA, Dedivitis RA, Pfuetzenreiter EG, Barros AP, dos Santos Queija D. Videolaryngostroboscopy and voice evaluation in patients with rheumatoid arthritis. Brazil Otorhinolaryngol. 2012;78(5):121–7.
16. Kırgezen T, Sünter AV, Yiğit Ö, Araz Server E, Aytekin E, Akar N, Sayıner Çağlar N. Influence disease activity on voice and laryngeal findings of rheumatoid arthritis patients. J Voice. 2020;34(3):451–5.
17. Bates CP. Proc Roy Soc Med. 1958;57(333):34.
18. Kolman J, Morris I. Cricoarytenoid arthritis: a cause of acute upper airway obstruction in rheumatoid arthritis. Canad J Anaesthe. 2002;49(7):729–93.
19. Pradhan P, Bhardwaj A, Venkatachalam VP. Bilateral cricoarytenoid arthritis: a cause of recurrent upper airway obstruction in rheumatoid arthritis. Malaysian J Med Sci. 2016;23(3):89.
20. Kosztyła-Hojna B, Moskal D, Kuryliszyn-Moskal A. Parameters of the assessment of voice quality and clinical manifestation of rheumatoid arthritis. Adv Med Sci. 2015;60(2):321–8.
21. Jurik AG, Pedersen U, Nøorgård A. Rheumatoid arthritis of the cricoarytenoid joints: a case of laryngeal obstruction due to acute and chronic joint changes. Laryngoscope. 1985;95(7 Pt 1):846–8.
22. Meng X, Xu HJ, Li RL, Zhao LD. Vocal cord lesions in representative autoimmune diseases. Clin Rheumatol. 2023;42(3):929–39.
23. Leicht MJ, Harrington TM, Davis DE. Cricoarytenoid arthritis: a cause of laryngeal obstruction. Ann Emerg Med. 1987;16(8):885–8.
24. Friedman BA. Rheumatoid nodules of the larynx. Arch Otolaryngol. 1975;101(6):361–3.
25. Woo P, Mendelsohn J, Humphrey D. Rheumatoid nodules of the larynx. Otolaryngol Head Neck Surg. 1995;113(1):147–50.
26. Hosako Y, Nakamura M, Tayama N, et al. Laryngeal involvements in systemic lupus erythematosus: a case report. Larynx Jpn. 1993;5:171–5.
27. Hilgert E, Toleti B, Kruger K, Nejedlo I. Hoarseness due to bamboo nodes in patients with autoimmune diseases: a review of literature. J Voice. 2008;22(3):343–50.

28. Applbaum E, Lichtbroun A. Novel Sjögren's autoantibodies found in fibromyalgia patients with sicca and/or xerostomia. Autoimmun Rev. 2019;18(2):199–202.
29. Shiboski CH, Shiboski SC, Seror R, et al. International Sjögren's syndrome criteria working group. 2016 American college of rheumatology/European league against rheumatism classification criteria for primary Sjögren's syndrome: a consensus and data-driven methodology involving three international patient cohorts. Arthritis Rheumatol. 2017;69(1):35–45.
30. Atzeni F, Cazzola M, Benucci M, Di Franco M, Salaffi F, Sarzi-Puttini P. Chronic widespread pain in the spectrum of rheumatological diseases. Best Pract Res Clin Rheumatol. 2011;25(2):165–71.
31. Gau SY, Leong PY, Lin CL, Tsou HK, Wei JC. Higher risk for Sjögren's syndrome in patients with fibromyalgia: a nationwide population-based cohort study. Front Immunol. 2021;12:640618.
32. Smets EM, Garssen B, Bonke B, De Haes JC. The Multidimensional Fatigue Inventory (MFI) psychometric qualities of an instrument to assess fatigue. J Psychosom Res. 1995;39:315–25.
33. d'Elia HF, Rehnberg E, Kvist G, Ericsson A, Konttinen Y, Mannerkorpi K. Fatigue and blood pressure in primary Sjogren's syndrome. Scand J Rheumatol. 2008;37(4):284–92.
34. Wolfe F, Clauw DJ, Fitzcharles MA, Goldenberg DL, Katz RS, Mease P, Russell AS, Russell IJ, Winfield JB, Yunus MB. The American college of rheumatology preliminary diagnostic criteria for fibromyalgia and measurement of symptom severity. Arthritis Care Res (Hoboken). 2010;62(5):600–10.
35. Choi BY, Oh HJ, Lee YJ, Song YW. Prevalence and clinical impact of fibromyalgia in patients with primary Sjögren's syndrome. Clin Exp Rheumatol. 2016;34(2 Suppl 96):S9–13.
36. Dubost JJ, Couderc M, Pereira B, et al. Concomitant fibromyalgia in primary Sjögren's syndrome in the French ASSESS cohort: comparison of the ACR 1990 and ACR 2016 criteria, FiRST questionnaire and physician's opinion. Clin Exp Rheumatol. 2021;39(Suppl 133(6)):140–5.
37. Wolfe F, Clauw DJ, Fitzcharles MA, Goldenberg DL, Häuser W, Katz RL, Mease PJ, Russell AS, Russell IJ, Walitt B. 2016 Revisions to the 2010/2011 fibromyalgia diagnostic criteria. Semin Arthritis Rheum. 2016;46(3):319–29.
38. Perrot S, Bouhassira D, Fermanian J. CEDR (Cercle d'Etude de la Douleur en Rhumatologie). Development and validation of the Fibromyalgia Rapid Screening Tool (FiRST). Pain. 2010;150(2):250–6.
39. Saghiri MA, Vakhnovetsky A, Vakhnovetsky J. Scoping review of the relationship between xerostomia and voice quality. Eur Arch Otorrinolaringol. 2023;280(7):3087–95.
40. Pierce JL, Tanner K, Merrill RM, Miller KL, Ambati BK, Kendall KA, Roy N. Voice disorders in Sjögren's syndrome: prevalence and related risk factors. Laryngoscope. 2015;125(6):1385–92.
41. Saltürk Z, Özdemir E, Kumral TL, Karabacakoğlu Z, Kumral E, Yildiz HF, Mersinlioğlu G, Atar Y, Berkiten G, Yildirim G, Uyar Y. Subjective and objective voice evaluation in Sjögren's syndrome. Logoped Phoniatr Vocol. 2017;42(1):9–11.
42. Heller A, Tanner K, Roy N, Nissen SL, Merrill RM, Miller KL, Houtz DR, Ellerston J, Kendall K. Voice, speech, and laryngeal features of primary Sjögren's syndrome. Ann Otol Rhinol Laryngol. 2014;123(11):778–85.
43. Zou ZF, Chen W, Li W, Yuan K. Impact of vocal fold dehydration on vocal function and its treatment. Current Medical Science. 2019;39:310–6.
44. Solomon NP. Vocal fatigue and its relation to vocal hyperfunction. Int J Speech Lang Pathol. 2008;10(4):254–66.
45. Sivasankar M, Erickson E, Schneider S, Hawes A. Phonatory effects of airway dehydration: preliminary evidence for impaired compensation to oral breathing in individuals with a history of vocal fatigue. J Speech Lang Hear Res. 2008;51(6):1494–506.
46. Sivasankar MP, Erickson-Levendoski E. Influence of obligatory mouth breathing, during realistic activities, on voice measures. J Voice. 2012;26(6):813.e9–13.
47. Hira D, Koshiyama S, Komase Y, Hoshino N, Morita SY, Terada T. Dry mouth as a novel indicator of hoarseness caused by inhalation therapy. J Asthma. 2015;52(3):296–300.

48. Lee JS, Keum BR, Kim JE, Park IS, Kim H. Prevalence of dysphonia in children with adenotonsillar problems and the impact of surgery on voice. Laryngoscope. 2021;131(10):2369–75.
49. Hamdan AL, Sibai A, Rameh C. Effect of fasting on voice in women. J Voice. 2007;21(4):495–501.
50. Alves M, Krüger E, Pillay B, Van Lierde K, Van der Linde J. The effect of hydration on voice quality in adults: a systematic review. J Voice. 2019;33(1):125–e13.
51. Sève P, Poupart M, Bui-Xuan C, Charhon A, Broussolle C. Cricoarytenoid arthritis in Sjögren's syndrome. Rheumatol Int. 2005;25(4):301–2.
52. Ito K, Yuyama S, Yamashita K, Hiiragi K, Tsukuda M, Ohishi K. A case report of Sjögren's syndrome with repeated false cord swelling. ORL J Otorhinolaryngol Relat Spec. 1994;56(3):173–6.
53. Prytz S. Vocal nodules in Sjögren's syndrome. J Laryngol Otol. 1980;94(2):197–203.
54. Todic J, Schweizer V, Leuchter I. Bamboo nodes of vocal folds: a description of 10 cases and review of the literature. Folia Phoniatr Logop. 2018;70(1):1–7.
55. Hanai S, Sato T, Akiyama Y, Nagatani K, Nagashima T, Iwamoto M, Kanazawa T, Minota S. Unilateral bamboo node of the vocal fold associated with anti-SS-A and anti-SS-B antibody. Auris Nasus Larynx. 2020;47(4):706–10.
56. Di Franco M, Guzzo MP, Spinelli FR, Atzeni F, Sarzi-Puttini P, Conti F, Iannuccelli C. Pain and systemic lupus erythematosus. Reumatismo. 2014;66(1):33–8.
57. Mistry S, Daoud A, Magrey MN, Pamuk ON. The frequency of fibromyalgia in patients with systemic lupus erythematosus and associated factors: a systematic review and meta-analysis. Clin Rheumatol. 2024;44:9–21.
58. Staud R. Are patients with systemic lupus erythematosus at increased risk for fibromyalgia? Curr Rheumatol Rep. 2006;8(6):430–5.
59. Middleton GD, McFarlin JE, Lipsky PE. The prevalence and clinical impact of fibromyalgia in systemic lupus erythematosus. Arthritis Rheum. 1994;37(8):1181–8.
60. Song Y, Kirsch G, Jarjour W. The utility of ultrasound in evaluating joint pain in systemic lupus erythematosus: looking beyond fibromyalgia. J Pers Med. 2023;13(5):763.
61. Kötter I, Neuscheler D, Günaydin I, Wernet D, Klein R. Is there a predisposition for the development of autoimmune diseases in patients with fibromyalgia? Retrospective analysis with long term follow-up. Rheumatol Int. 2007;27(11):1031–9.
62. Murano E, Hosako-Naito Y, Tayama N, Oka T, Miyaji M, Kumada M, Niimi S. Bamboo node: primary vocal fold lesion as evidence of autoimmune disease. J Voice. 2001;15(3):441–50.
63. Lee JH, Sung IY, Park JH, Roh JL. Recurrent laryngeal neuropathy in a systemic lupus erythematosus (SLE) patient. Am J Phys Med Rehabil. 2008;87(1):68–70.
64. Leszczynski P, Pawlak-Bus K. Vocal cords palsy in systemic lupus erythematosus patient: diagnostic and therapeutic difficulties. Rheumatol Int. 2013;33(6):1577–80.
65. de Macedo MSFC, Costa KM, da Silva Filho M. Voice disorder in systemic lupus erythematosus. PLoS One. 2017;12(4):e0175893.
66. Golder V, Schachna L. Ankylosing spondylitis: an update. Aust Fam Physician. 2013;42(11):780–4.
67. Jethwa H, Bowness P. The interleukin (IL)-23/IL-17 axis in ankylosing spondylitis: new advances and potentials for treatment. Clin Exp Immunol. 2016;183(1):30–6.
68. Simone D, Al Mossawi MH, Bowness P. Progress in our understanding of the pathogenesis of ankylosing spondylitis. Rheumatology (Oxford). 2018;57(Suppl_6):vi4–9.
69. Aloush V, Ablin JN, Reitblat T, Caspi D, Elkayam O. Fibromyalgia in women with ankylosing spondylitis. Rheumatol Int. 2007;27(9):865–8.
70. Calin A, Garrett S, Whitelock H, Kennedy LG, O'Hea J, Mallorie P, Jenkinson T. A new approach to defining functional ability in ankylosing spondylitis: the development of the bath ankylosing spondylitis functional index. J Rheumatol. 1994;21(12):2281–5.
71. Almodóvar R, Carmona L, Zarco P, Collantes E, González C, Mulero J, Sueiro JL, Gratacós J, Torre-Alonso JC, Juanola X, Batlle E, Ariza R, Font P. Fibromyalgia in patients with ankylosing spondylitis: prevalence and utility of the measures of activity, function and radiological damage. Clin Exp Rheumatol. 2010;28(6 Suppl 63):S33–9.

72. Baraka E, Balata M, Ahmed S, El-Blbehisy M, Elattar E. Concomitant diagnosis of fibromyalgia and ankylosing spondylitis: relation to clinical features and plasma pentraxin −3 level. Curr Rheumatol Rev. 2021;17(3):331–41.
73. Gau SY, Lee YH, Tsou HK, Huang JY, Chen X, Ye Z, Wei JC. Patients with ankylosing spondylitis are associated with high risk of fibromyalgia: a nationwide population-based cohort study. Front Med. 2021;8:618594.
74. Ahmed EA, Atar S, Atar Y, Sari H, Anarat MEA, Saltürk Z, Karaketir SG, Uyar Y, Kuru Ö. Evaluation of the swallowing and voice functions in ankylosing spondylitis patients. Dysphagia. 2022;37(2):455–62.
75. Bienenstock H, Lanyi VF. Cricoarytenoid arthritis in a patient with ankylosing spondylitis. Arch Otolaryngol. 1977;103(12):738–9.
76. Miller FR, Wanamaker JR, Hicks DM, Tucker HM. Cricoarytenoid arthritis and ankylosing spondylitis. Arch Otolaryngol Head Neck Surg. 1994;120(2):214–6.
77. Erdogmus B, Yazici B, Ozturk O, Ataoglu S, Yazici S. Laryngocele in association with ankylosing spondylitis. Wien Klin Wochenschr. 2005;117(19–20):718–20.
78. Jang S, Lee K, Ju JH. Recent updates of diagnosis, pathophysiology, and treatment on osteoarthritis of the knee. Int J Mol Sci. 2021;22(5):2619.
79. Xia B, Chen D, Zhang J, Hu S, Jin H, Tong P. Osteoarthritis pathogenesis: a review of molecular mechanisms. Calcif Tissue Int. 2014;95(6):495–505.
80. Mahgoub MY, Elnady BM, Abdelkader HS, Abdelhalem RA, Hassan WA. Comorbidity of fibromyalgia in primary knee osteoarthritis: potential impact on functional status and quality of life. Open Access Rheumatol. 2020;12:55–63.
81. Bernatsky S, Dobkin PL, Penrod JR, De C. Co-morbidity and physician use in fibromyalgia. Swiss Med Wkly. 2005;135(0506):76.
82. Haviland MG, Banta JE, Przekop P. Fibromyalgia: prevalence, course, and co-morbidities in hospitalized patients in the United States, 1999–2007. Clin Exp Rheumatol. 2011;29(6 Suppl 69):S79–87.
83. Paulsen FP, Tillmann BN. Osteoarthritis in cricoarytenoid joint. Osteoarthr Cartil. 1999;7(6):505–14.
84. Virk JS, Majithia A, Lingam RK, Singh A. Cervical osteophytes causing vocal fold paralysis: case report and literature review. J Laryngol Otol. 2012;126(9):963–5.

Pain, Central Sensitization in Fibromyalgia and Voice

9

Abdul-latif Hamdan, Robert Thayer Sataloff, and Mary J. Hawkshaw

The Neurobiology of Pain in Fibromyalgia

Pain is defined as "an unpleasant sensory and emotional experience associated with, actual or potential tissue damage or described in terms of such damage" [1]. It is a global health issue associated with an increase in comorbidities, decrease in quality of life, and with premature death [2]. Different types of pain mechanisms have been described including nociceptive pain which relates to the somatosensory system, neuropathic pain which relates to damage to the nervous system, and nociplastic pain that refers to dysfunction in pain processing. Peripheral nociceptors involved in pain processing include the C fibers, A delta fibers and A beta fibers, each having different noxious stimuli and thresholds. For instance, the C fibers are activated by low threshold thermal, chemical or mechanical stimuli and carry the input to Lamina II in the spinal cord dorsal horn (SCDH), whereas A delta fibers are activated by low intensity mechanical stimuli and carry the input to lamina III-IV of the SCDH. The ascending pain pathways originating from the SCDH, namely the spinothalamic, spinomesencephalic and spinoreticular tracts, decussate in the spinal cord before reaching multiple pain processing areas in the brain [2, 3].

Musculoskeletal diseases, including Fibromyalgia, account for a large percentage of chronic pain conditions. Fibromyalgia is characterized by chronic pain and body fatigue associated with a myriad of somatic and non-somatic symptoms that cause adverse effects on the physical and psychological well-being of affected patients [4]. The pain in FM is very complex and multidimensional. It has both a central and peripheral component and is considered by many as nociplastic in nature. The use of functional magnetic resonance imaging and other techniques such as spectroscopy has allowed scientists and researchers to gain more insights on the pathophysiology of pain in FM. The current literature carries strong evidence that FM patients suffer from alteration in pain processing in two major central areas

A.-l. Hamdan et al., *Voice Disorders in Fibromyalgia*,
https://doi.org/10.1007/978-3-031-97751-0_9

in the brain, the sensory-discriminative network and the affective and emotional network. The former includes the somatosensory cortices I and II, the lateral nuclei of the thalamus and the posterior insula cortex, whereas the latter includes the anterior insula cortex, the medial thalamic nuclei and the amygdala. Other areas in the brain including the limbic system also are engaged in pain processing. In patients with FM, there is alteration in this complex network of pain processing in these various regions in the brain, and the aberrations in pain processing occur both at rest and during pain stimulation [5–9]. This aberration has been shown to be coupled with an imbalance in neurotransmitters and neuromodulators. Spectroscopic studies have shown the presence of molecular changes in the pain processing areas, namely an imbalance between the excitatory neurotransmitters and the inhibitory ones. An example is the increase in the ratio of glutamate to y-aminobutyric acid (GABA) [10–12].

In addition to the central sensitization, there is also dysfunction in the descending inhibitory systems that are partially responsible for modulating the perception of pain. Numerous studies have shown that the analgesic effect known as “diffuse noxious inhibitory control” responsible for whole-body analgesia following the application of a strong painful stimulus is reduced in FM patients [13, 14]. In other words, the balance between the excitatory and inhibitory control of pain is disturbed with overwhelming of the excitatory component. Suggested mechanisms include alteration in secretion of serotonin and its precursors, among other neurotransmitters [14]. Other suggested mechanisms for pain in FM include disturbance in the hypothalamic-pituitary axis and small fiber neuropathy [15, 16]. Readers can refer to Chap. 4 on the pathophysiology of FM, and Chap. 10 on muscle dysfunction for more information.

The neurobiology of pain in FM is complex. The main pathophysiology is alteration in the pain processing areas in two main networks in the brain, the affective emotional network and the sensory discriminative network. Disturbance in these networks has been linked to an imbalance in the neurotransmitters and neuromodulators resulting in dominance of the excitatory component. Dysfunction in the descending inhibitory pathway for pain control has accentuated pain perception further in affected patients. Future research on the interplay between the central and peripheral etiologies of pain is needed to elucidate better treatment strategies.

Impact of Pain on Voice in FM Patients

It is well established that the human voice conveys non-verbal expressions similar to those conveyed by facial and/or body gestures. In addition to being an acoustic cue to age and gender, voice conveys signs of health and well-being and expresses a myriad of positive and negative emotions. Common examples of overt emotional vocalizations are laughter, cry, sigh, screams and grunts in response to painful or pleasant stimuli, all of which add to linguistic communication and to the more subtle emotional content of speech. Many studies have shown that these non-linguistic emotional sounds are recognized with accuracy that exceeds chance despite cultural differences, thus making voice a universal para-verbal messenger that transcends cultural and linguistic variations [17, 18].

The role of emotional vocal sounds as a universal language is gaining interest, as these sounds surpass linguistic and cultural barriers. The distinguished acoustic features of different non-verbal sounds produced that allow the listener to discern between different emotional vocalizations are intriguing. In a review of acoustic features of positive emotions, *Kamiloglu et al.* noted that in state of arousal such as anger and happiness, there is an increase in pitch and loudness. In happiness, there is also increase in pitch range and variability, as well as an increase in the first two formants. When compared with other positive emotions, the fundamental frequency in happiness was found to be higher [17]. Emotional vocalization of sounds indicative of pain are also perceived differently. As a result of biopsychological stimuli and as an adaptive process to a painful event, vocalizations have been shown to be indicators of pain and to have distinctive acoustic features. Although these have scarcely been investigated, most studies agree that with pain there is an increase in pitch and loudness similar to what has been reported in other emotions such as distress [19, 20]. *Lautenbacher et al.* investigated the phonetic characteristics of four vowels vocalized during painful and non-painful conditions. Fifty students were asked to produce the vowels /u/, /ɑ/, /i/ and /ə/ while their hands were immersed in water tanks the temperature of which varied from 41 to 47 Celsius. The participants were also asked to rate their pain using Numerical Rating Scales. The results showed that thermal stimulation had a significant effect on the pitch of /u/ and /ə/ and on loudness of /schwa/. Both loudness and pitch increased for /schwa/ during painful stimulation [21]. *Anikin and Person* introduced a corpus of 260 non-linguistic vocalization that included all types of emotions as well pain, and validated these vocalizations by asking listeners to recognize the type of emotions. The recognition accuracy for pain was less than 40%, whereas the recognition accuracy for amusement, fear, sadness, amusement and pleasure exceeded 70%. The most reliable acoustic predictors of these non-linguistic vocalizations were voice pitch, spacing of syllables and harmonicity. The cultural background of listeners had no impact on recognition accuracy. The audio clips evaluated by listeners were taken from online videos [18]. Icht et al. investigated the role of vocal expressions of intellectually disabled individuals as indicators of pain and noted that pain-related vocalization had more number of pulses, i.e., segment that contained clear harmonic structure consistent with phonation, and had higher shimmer value. The study was conducted on nine subjects using acoustic analysis of spontaneous vocal expressions, namely vowel-like sounds such as yelling, crying and moaning. The authors suggested these may be used as indicators of pain in disabled patients who cannot speak [22]. *Pisanski et al.* investigated whether the fundamental frequency (F0) remains an acoustic cue to the speaker identity across non-verbal vocalizations including pain. The authors noted a correlation between the fundamental frequency (F0) and intensity of pain. The mean F0 for mild pain vocalization was 465 Hz whereas for intense pain it was 738 Hz. The results also indicated that individual differences in F0 were retained across all different non-verbal vocalizations including those in response to pain [23].

The acoustic properties of cry response to painful stimuli in children have also been of interest for physicians and non-physicians. The cry of infants and neonates has been used as an indicator of extent of pain during various interventions. *Porter et al.* in their descriptive neural model of cry production, noted that the cry of chronically ill infants had a higher pitch than that of healthy infants. The authors also reported an increase in the infants' cries in association with a decrease in vagal tone. This latter was measured using heart rate and amplitude of respiratory sinus arrhythmia [24]. *Fuller BF,* investigated the acoustic properties of three different types of cries in 2–4-month-old infants and noted that procedural pain-related cries and hungry-related cries were more tense than fussy cries, and procedural pain-induced cries had higher second formant amplitudes than hungry cries and fussy cries [25]. *Grunau et al.* conducted acoustic analysis of cry in 36 full-term infants who underwent three types of procedures. Of the 36 babies, all but two cried following injection, 16 cried following alcohol swab to the alternate thigh, and 11 cried following application of triple dye to the umbilical cord. Eight babies cried following all three stimuli. The authors noted significant difference in latency and duration of cry across these procedures. The latency of cry was shorter and the duration of cry was longer during injection in comparison to the cry of those who underwent alcohol swabs and dye application to the umbilical cord. There was no significant difference in jitter or melody. The authors concluded that cry activity may be used as an indicator of degree of pain during invasive procedures [26].

Artificial intelligence and machine learning techniques are being used to detect pain in vocal expressions. Both acute and chronic pain are being detected with high accuracy using multiple artificial neural networks [27]. In a study to improve triage classification of pain, *Tsai et al.* proposed a model that relies on facial and vocal expressions detected from audio-visual recordings of patients. The proposed framework achieved an accuracy of 72.3% [28].

How can pain impact voice? Pain can impact voice by causing alterations in any of the components of the phonatory system. Pain in the cervical region for instance can extend to the laryngeal muscles and result in heightened tension and deviant phonatory behavior. Similarly, distant body aches like low back pain may lead to excess tension in the posterior cervical muscles as noted by *Rubin et al.* [29]. The authors described the term "equipoise" in reference to the ideal body posture where the head is fully aligned vertically with the rest of the body [29]. A disturbance in this alignment can lead to overpowering of the posterior deep neck extensor muscles resulting in an increase in laryngeal muscle tension. This notion of synergy between the cervical muscles, posture and phonatory apparatus has been also asserted by *Cielo et al.* in their review on musculoskeletal stress syndrome [30]. The motor adjustment in the cervical muscles as a result of low back pain and poor posture can lead to hyperfunction in the laryngeal muscles and in increase in mechanical stress. Titze et al. noted collision between the vocal folds is a main mechanical stress factors in phonation [31]. Excess tension in the laryngeal muscles and acceleration in the collision force can lead to tissue damage and predispose to structural voice disorders [33].

At the level of the power source, numerous studies indicate that pain has an adverse effect on breathing. Sataloff R.T in his review on the work-up and examination of patients with voice disorders, stressed the paramount importance of a good posture in phonation and the its intricate role in breathing particularly in professional voice users [32, 33]. Low back pain may impair the activity of the respiratory muscles and jeopardize maximum inspiratory and expiratory capacity. *Shah et al.* examined the respiratory function of 14 patients with chronic lower back pain and found significantly lower mean maximum voluntary ventilation and higher mean end-tidal Carbon Dioxide (PETCO2) in comparison to 14 healthy subjects. However, this difference became non-significant when adjusting for gender as a variable [34]. *Rasouli et al.* investigated abdominal muscle activity using ultrasound imaging in 18 patients with low back pain while performing three sitting positions (on a chair, on a gym ball, on a gym ball with the left foot raised). Except for the external obliques, patients had a decrease in activity of the abdominal muscles during respiration when sitting on a gym ball and lifting their left foot [35] These findings suggest that professional voice users with chronic low back pain cannot use their abdominal muscles efficiently while performing vocally demanding tasks [36]. Pain in the cervical region has also been linked to a decrease in respiratory capacity. *Kapreli et al.* investigated respiratory function in 12 patients with chronic neck pain and found a significant decrease in maximal voluntary ventilation and respiratory muscle strength in comparison to healthy controls. The authors also noted an association between the decrease in respiratory muscle strength and forward head posture [36]. Last but not least, pain may also affect voice by altering the shape and configuration of the resonators. A common example is temporomandibular dysfunction. Affected patients may present with vocal symptoms as a result of limited range of movement of the temporomandibular joint [32, 33]. Adessa et al. conducted an investigation on the association between TMJ dysfunction and voice-related quality of life and noted that the majority, 80% of the study group, had some form of impairement, although minimal. The authors advocated a multidisciplinary approach in the treatment of patients with TMJ dysfunction [37].

Chronic pain may also impact phonation as a result of stress and mental disturbance. Patients with chronic pain suffer from an increase in emotional liability and are at a high risk of having anxiety and depression. *Krishan et al.* examined the association between depression and chronic pain and noted major and minor depression in 31 and 8 out 71 patients with chronic pain. Additionally, 18 participants had intermittent depressive disorder [38]. *Elliot et al.* investigated the link between depression and chronic pain in 160 women and noted major depressive symptoms in 52% of the cases. Moreover, there was a correlation between depression and the SF-36 score [39]. That said, it is also well established that mental illnesses have adverse effect on phonation. Patients with anxiety and depression are at higher risk of having voice disorders than healthy subjects with no mental illnesses. The reader can refer to Chap. 13 of this book for further reference.

There is substantial evidence that vocalization of pain, similar to other type of negative and positive emotional vocalizations, has distinctive acoustic features. The most commonly described are increase in pitch and loudness. In infants, there is also an increase in the first two formants. Suggested mechanisms for the change in voice quality in patients with pain include alteration laryngeal muscle tension and dysfunction in the respiratory system.

References

1. International Association for the Study of Pain. Terminology; 2021. https://www.iasp-pain.org/Education/Content.aspx?ItemNumber=1698#Pain.
2. Mills SE, Nicolson KP, Smith BH. Chronic pain: a review of its epidemiology and associated factors in population-based studies. Br J Anaesth. 2019;123:e273–83.
3. Al-Khater KM, Todd AJ. Collateral projections of neurons in laminae I, III, and IV of rat spinal cord to thalamus, periaqueductal gray matter, and lateral parabrachial area. J Comp Neurol. 2009;515:629–46.
4. Favretti M, Iannuccelli C, Di Franco M. Pain biomarkers in fibromyalgia syndrome: current understanding and future directions. Int J Mol Sci. 2023;24(13):10443.
5. Vachon-Presseau E, Tétreault P, Petre B, et al. Corticolimbic anatomical characteristics predetermine risk for chronic pain. Brain J Neurol. 2016;139:1958–70.
6. Bolwerk A, Seifert F, Maihöfner C. Altered resting-state functional connectivity in complex regional pain syndrome. J Pain. 2013;14:1107–15.
7. Letzen JE, Robinson ME. Negative mood influences default mode network functional connectivity in patients with chronic low back pain: implications for functional neuroimaging biomarkers. Pain. 2017;158:48–57.
8. Loggia ML, Kim J, Gollub RL, et al. Default mode network connectivity encodes clinical pain: an arterial spin labeling study. Pain. 2013;154:24–33.
9. Baliki MN, Apkarian AV. Nociception, pain, negative moods, and behavior selection. Neuron. 2015;87:474–91.
10. Foerster BR, Petrou M, Edden RA, et al. Reduced insular γ-aminobutyric acid in fibromyalgia. Arthritis Rheum. 2012;64:579–83.
11. Pyke TL, Osmotherly PG, Baines S. Measuring glutamate levels in the brains of fibromyalgia patients and a potential role for glutamate in the pathophysiology of fibromyalgia symptoms: a systematic review. Clin J Pain. 2017;33:944–54.
12. Emmer BJ, van der Bijl AE, Huizinga TW, et al. Brain involvement in rheumatoid arthritis: a magnetic resonance spectroscopy study. Arthritis Rheum. 2009;60:3190–5.
13. Kosek E, Hansson P. Modulatory influence on somatosensory perception from vibration and Heterotopic Noxious Conditioning Stimulation (HNCS) in fibromyalgia patients and healthy subjects. Pain. 1997;70(1):41–51.
14. Julien N, Marchand S. Endogenous pain inhibitory systems activated by spatial summation are opioid-mediated. Neurosci Lett. 2006;401(3):256–60.
15. Russell IJ, Michalek JE, Vipraio GA, Fletcher EM, Javors MA, Bowden CA. Platelet 3H-imipramine uptake receptor density and serum serotonin levels in patients with fibromyalgia/fibrositis syndrome. J Rheumatol. 1992;19(1):104–9.
16. Pérez-Neri I, Sandoval H, Estêvão MD, Vasanthan LT, Alarcon-Ruiz CA, Ruszkowski J, Mathangasinghe Y, Ríos C, Pineda C. Central and peripheral mechanisms of pain in fibromyalgia: scoping review protocol. Rheumatol Int. 2023;43(4):757–62.
17. Kamiloğlu RG, Fischer AH, Sauter DA. Good vibrations: a review of vocal expressions of positive emotions. Psychon Bull Rev. 2020;27(2):237–65.
18. Anikin A, Persson T. Nonlinguistic vocalizations from online amateur videos for emotion research: a validated corpus. Behav Res Methods. 2017;49(2):758–71.
19. Pisanski K, Bryant GA. The evolution of voice perception. In: The oxford handbook of voice studies. Oxford University Press; 2019. p. 269–300.

20. Ryalls JH, Lieberman P. Fundamental frequency and vowel perception. J Acoust Soc Am. 1982;72(5):1631–4.
21. Lautenbacher S, Salinas-Ranneberg M, Niebuhr O, Kunz M. Phonetic characteristics of vocalizations during pain. Pain Rep. 2017;2(3):e597.
22. Icht M, Wiznitser Ressis-tal H, Lotan M. Can the vocal expression of intellectually disabled individuals be used as a pain indicator? Initial findings supporting a possible novice assessment method. Front Psychol. 2021;12:655202.
23. Pisanski K, Raine J, Reby D. Individual differences in human voice pitch are preserved from speech to screams, roars and pain cries. R Soc Open Sci. 2020;7(2):191642.
24. Porter FL, Porges SW, Marshall RE. Newborn pain cries and vagal tone: parallel changes in response to circumcision. Child Dev. 1988;59(2):495–505.
25. Fuller BF. Acoustic discrimination of three types of infant cries. Nurs Res. 1991;40(3):156–60.
26. Grunau RVE, Johnston CC, Craig KD. Neonatal facial and cry responses to invasive and non-invasive procedures. Pain. 1990;42(3):295–305.
27. Borna S, Haider CR, Maita KC, Torres RA, Avila FR, Garcia JP, De Sario Velasquez GD, McLeod CJ, Bruce CJ, Carter RE, Forte AJ. A review of voice-based pain detection in adults using artificial intelligence. Bioengineering. 2023;10(4):500.
28. Tsai FS, Hsu YL, Chen WC, Weng YM, Ng CJ, Lee CC. Toward development and evaluation of pain level-rating scale for emergency triage based on vocal characteristics and facial expressions. In: Interspeech. ISCA; 2016. p. 92–6.
29. Rubin JS, Blake E, Mathieson L. Musculoskeletal patterns in patients with voice disorders. J Voice. 2007;21(4):477–84.
30. Cielo CA, Christmann MK, Ribeiro VV, Hoffmann CF, Padilha JF, Steidl EM, Bastilha GR, Andriollo DB, Frigo LF. Musculoskeletal stress syndrome, extrinsic laryngeal muscles and body posture: theoretical considerations. Revista CEFAC. 2014;16:1639–49.
31. Titze IR. Mechanical stress in phonation. J Voice. 1994;8(2):99–105.
32. Sataloff RT. Patient history. In: Sataloff RT, editor. The professional voice. 4th ed. San Diego: Plural Publishing; 2017. p. 363–87.
33. Sataloff RT. Physical examination. In: Sataloff RT, editor. The professional voice. 4th ed. San Diego: Plural Publishing; 2017. p. 391–405.
34. Shah SG, Choezom T, Raja GP. Comparison of respiratory parameters in participants with and without chronic low back pain. J Bodyw Mov Ther. 2019;23(4):894–900.
35. Rasouli O, Shanbehzadeh S, Arab AM, ShahAli S, Sarafraz H. The effect of respiratory phase on abdominal muscle activity during stable and unstable sitting positions in individuals with and without chronic low back pain. J Manip Physiol Ther. 2020;43(3):225–33.
36. Kapreli E, Vourazanis E, Billis E, Oldham JA, Strimpakos N. Respiratory dysfunction in chronic neck pain patients. A pilot study. Cephalalgia. 2009;29(7):701–10.
37. Adessa M, Kim J, Tierney WS, Benninger M. Temporomandibular dysfunction and voice related quality of life impairment. Laryngoscope. 2024;134(1):315–7.
38. Krishnan KR, France RD, Pelton S, McCann UD, Davidson J, Urban BJ. Chronic pain and depression. I. Classification of depression in chronic low back pain patients. Pain. 1985;22(3):279–87.
39. Elliott TE, Renier CM, Palcher JA. Chronic pain, depression, and quality of life: correlations and predictive value of the SF-36. Pain Med. 2003;4(4):331–9.

Impact of Reduced Muscle Strength in Fibromyalgia on Voice

10

Abdul-latif Hamdan, Robert Thayer Sataloff,
and Mary J. Hawkshaw

Prevalence of Muscle Dysfunction in Fibromyalgia (FM)

Patients with Fibromyalgia (FM) present with diffuse and persistent muscle pain of at least 3 months duration. The muscle pain often is associated with body fatigue, stiffness, and decrease in activity. Numerous authors have shown that muscle symptoms in FM are secondary not only to central sensitization and alteration in pain processing but also to muscle dysfunction. This mechanism is substantiated by numerous reports on reduced muscle strength, decrease in voluntary maximal muscle contraction and early exhaustion in FM patients. In 1987, *Jacobson and Danneskiold-Samsoe* measured the strength of knee extension in 15 patients with fibrositis syndrome, a term previously used to describe FM, and noted a reduction in maximal isometric strength by almost 60%, and in maximum isokinetic strength by almost 50% in comparison to healthy controls [1]. In 1990, *Mengshoel and Komnaes* tested 26 women diagnosed with FM and found lower strength in the upper extremities in comparison to controls (58 ± 22 kPa in FM vs. 97 ± 17 kPa, respectively). The dynamic and static endurance values also were reduced compared to healthy subjects. The dynamic endurance work was measured by asking the patient to perform repetitive maximal grip pressure, whereas the static endurance work was assessed by asking the patient to keep the upper extremities in a fixed position. The fatigue score based on the extent of perceived exertion was significantly higher (worse) in patients with FM in comparison to controls [2]. In 1993, *Nordenskiold and Grimby* investigated the grip force of 51 right-handed women, 14 of whom had FM, and found a decrease by almost 40% in the FM group compared to the control group. The ratio of average force to peak force over the course of 10 s was 69% in patients with FM in comparison to 83% in healthy women [3]. In 1994, *Lindh et al.* examined muscle contraction in 25

A.-l. Hamdan et al., *Voice Disorders in Fibromyalgia*,
https://doi.org/10.1007/978-3-031-97751-0_10

patients with FM and found a reduction in strength of knee flexion and extension in comparison to 22 healthy controls. Superimposed electrical stimulation improved the muscle performance indicating that the maximal voluntary muscle contraction was decreased and not all the motor units were recruited. Seventy-nine percent of the FM group had a submaximal torque voluntarily versus only one out of ten in the control group. The reduced maximal muscle contraction was noted in isometric, isokinetic and eccentric tests. For example, the maximal voluntary isometric torque in extension was 56% of the value obtained in controls. Similarly, in flexion, the value was 53% of that of the control group. The authors discussed the possible reasons for the decreased voluntary muscle contraction and alluded to central impairment as a possible cause. Other potential causes included a decrease in motivation, as well as pain and/or fear of pain [4]. In 1995, *Norregaard et al.* reported lower quadriceps muscle strength per cross-sectional area in patients with FM in comparison to controls (91 Nm vs. 125 Nm, respectively). Furthermore, there was a reduction in muscle strength (voluntary) of the knee flexors and plantar flexors [5]. In 1997, *Norregaard et al.* evaluated the physical effort and capacity of 181 patients with FM and reported a 20%–30% reduction in voluntary muscle strength of the flexors and extensors of the knee and elbow. The decrease in performance could be attributed to the low degree of effort as evidenced by an increase in heart rate to only 63% of the predicted increase [6]. The author's argument is valid given that the cardiac muscles are not skeletal muscles and their involvement in FM has not been reported in the literature. In 2002, *Maquet et al.* examined the muscle performance in 16 women with FM and noted reduced maximal concentric isokinetic muscle strength, fatigue resistance and static endurance in comparison to 85 healthy controls by 39%, 40% and 81%, respectively. Impairment in muscle function was more prominent during aerobic exercise [7]. In 2012, *M Goes et al.* investigated lower limb muscle performance in 16 FM female patients and found a decrease in muscle strength, namely lower extension peak torque, in comparison to controls, and lower rate of torque development. Patients also had a decrease in hip adduction and in extension peak torque which were predictive of number of falls [8]. In 2020, *Mulkoglu et al.* investigated the isokinetic trunk muscle strength in 46 women with FM using an isokinetic dynamometer and found significantly lower values in trunk extensor peak torque values in comparison to controls [9]. In 2022, *Kapuczinski et al.* examined muscle function and sarcopenia in FM patients using validated questionnaires and bio-impedance analysis of muscle mass and handgrip strength. The results showed significantly higher scores (worse) and significantly lower muscle performance and strength in the FM group compared to controls. There was no significant difference in muscle mass between the two groups [10].

In summary, numerous studies indicate that FM is associated with muscle dysfunction that manifests as a decrease in isometric and isokinetic strength, in maximal voluntary contraction, and in endurance. When the lower limb muscles are affected, patients are at a higher risk for falls. Several mechanisms have been suggested, as discussed in the section below.

Suggested Mechanisms for Muscle Dysfunction in FM

The etiology of muscle dysfunction in FM is still unknown. Several hypotheses have been suggested, one of which is impaired oxygenation and mitochondrial dysfunction [11]. In a 2025 review of muscle dysfunction in FM, *Rubio-Zarapuz* showed ample evidence supporting the premise that a decrease in tissue oxygen uptake and utilization plays an etiologic role in FM [12]. This review concurred with numerous reports documenting impaired tissue oxygenation in FM patients. *Kaylan-Raman et al.* performed histochemical and electron microscopic examination of muscle biopsies taken from patients with FM and showed evidence of muscle fiber necrosis and glycogen deposition suggestive of ischemia [13]. *Lund al et* examined subcutaneous tissue oxygenation at trigger points in ten patients with FM and reported lower values in comparison to controls. The oxygen pressure was measured using a multipoint oxygen electrode that captured the variations in oxygenation in relation to capillary blood flow and hemoglobin oxygen affinity [14]. *Bengtsson et al.* investigated muscle energy metabolism of biopsies taken from painful sites in the trapezius muscle in 15 patients with FM and noted higher levels of creatinine and adenosine monophosphate (AMP), and lower levels of adenosine triphosphate (ATP), adenosine diphosphate (ADP) and phosphocreatine (PC) in comparison to biopsies taken from normal subjects. As decrease in these levels usually is observed following prolonged ischemia [15], the authors attributed their findings to hypoxia and metabolic changes that led to an increase in the degradation of energy-rich phosphates and/or a decrease in their synthesis. It is important to note that there was no significant difference between the biopsies taken from non-tender sites in FM patients and controls [16]. *Gerdle et al.* examined the blood flow and metabolic substances in the trapezius and erector spinae muscles and reported lower blood flow, lower phosphocreatinine and nucleotide triphosphate in erector spinae muscles of FM patients in comparison to healthy controls. The authors suggested mitochondrial dysfunction as a possible cause [17]. *Villafaina et al.* investigated oxygen consumption within quadriceps muscles of FM patients during a fatigue-task which consisted of repeated flexion and extension (n = 20 times) of the quadriceps. The authors reported lower muscle oxygen saturation in FM patients versus controls (56.03 + 21.36 vs. 77.41 + 10.82, respectively). Similarly, the oxygenated hemoglobin level was lower in comparison to healthy subjects (6.69 + 2.59 vs. 9.37 + 1.31, respectively) [18]. In 2024, *Inferrera et al.* examined mitochondrial dysfunction and level of oxidative stress in limb skeletal muscles of rats injected with reserpine to induce FM. The authors noted expression of oxidative stress markers along with impaired mobility of the limbs. Moreover, the injection of Boswellia serrata gum resin extract (BS) which is known to induce antioxidants, resulted in upregulation of mitochondrial function and the expression of antioxidants [19]. In a review on the link between muscle symptoms in FM, (pain and fatigue) and muscle oxygen saturation, *Rubio-Zarapuz et al.* highlighted the high prevalence of alteration in oxygen uptake and suboptimal utilization in muscle fibers both at rest and during activity. The increase in metabolic end products was believed to be partially responsible for the heightened pain and fatigue in affected patients. The authors highlighted that a decrease in microcirculation and impairment of in the structure and function of mitochondria may play an etiologic role [12].

Another suggested mechanism for muscle dysfunction in FM is degeneration of tissue secondary to chronic inflammation and microtrauma. Using electron microscopic examination, *Kaylan-Raman et al.* noted atrophic changes in type II fibers and moth-eaten appearance of type I fibers at trigger points in the trapezius muscle of patients with FM suggestive of chronic inflammatory changes [13]. *Bengtsson et al.* conducted a histopathological and histochemical examination of muscle biopsies taken from 57 patients diagnosed with FM and reported pathologic changes in 35 cases [20]. The most common were degeneration and regeneration consistent with a state of chronic inflammation. Although the presence of "moth-eaten" fibers was not diagnostic of Fibromyalgia, it was suggestive of ischemic changes [21]. *Umay et al.* evaluated muscle tissue of the upper and lower extremities of 102 patients with FM and noted a decrease in cross sectional area of the quadriceps femoris [22]. *Wang et al.* examined circulating cytokine levels over the course of 6 months in 20 patients with FM in comparison to 80 controls and found higher baseline level of IL-8 which corelated with the level of pain ($r = -0.782$), and high-level TNF-alpha. The elevated levels of IL-8 and TNF-alpha suggestive of an inflammatory process decreased following treatment [23].

Another possible cause of impaired muscle function is physical inactivity as a result of deconditioning associated with pain and disuse of skeletal muscles [24–26]. Physical inactivity may perpetuate disease-induced degenerative changes and promote muscle atrophy. *Vancampfort et al.* conducted a systematic review and meta-analysis on physical activity in FM patients and noted that the overall level was lower than what has been recommended in 63.3% of affected subjects. The majority were not active enough or engaged in the required physical activity to meet the health benefits of exercise [27]. In another systematic review, the same authors noted that pain intensity, physical and mental health, and lack of motivation were significant barriers that accentuated sedentary behavior [28]. *Karacay et al.* conducted a case-control study which included 107 patients with FM and found a positive correlation between kynophobia and fatigue. An increase in severity of pain led to more disability, fatigue and kinophobia, and vice-versa. The authors stressed the vicious cycle of body fatigue and fear of moving [29]. *Gutierrez et al.* examined functional disability in relation to chronic pain and fatigue in 76 women and found that avoiding pain influenced sedentarism and level of activity such as walking. The authors stressed the importance of addressing motivation to circumvent the pain-avoidance goals in FM patients [30].

The impact of stress and psychogenic state on muscle function in FM also has been investigated [31–34]. Many authors suggested that the decrease in voluntary muscle strength in patients with FM can be attributed to impairment in central drive and decrease in motivation as a result of anxiety and depression [35, 36]. In a review on depression and physical activity, *Bueno-antequera et al.* stressed on the adverse impact of the former on sedentary behavior and the important role of physical exercise in preventing depression. In their study, depressed people also had an increased risk of cardiovascular diseases type 2 diabetes, and they tended to have a shorter life [37]. *Gavilan-Carrera et al.* conducted a cross-sectional study on 386 women with FM and found an association between sedentary time and symptoms of depression and anxiety. The authors noted that physical fitness and exercise might help decrease those symptoms, although moderate-to-vigorous physical activity did not affect the correlation between sedentary time and those mental disorders [38].

There is more than one pathological mechanism potentially responsible for muscle dysfunction in FM. Several mechanisms have been suggested including alteration in metabolism, impaired oxygenation and mitochondrial dysfunction. The poor oxygenation of muscle tissue can be attributed to impairment in capillary perfusion as a result of intravascular narrowing. Other possible mechanisms include inactivity, fear of pain, kynophobia, and depression which all can act in concert to reduce motivation and the drive to exercise.

The Impact of Muscle Dysfunction on Voice in FM Patients

As discussed in Chap. 5, the prevalence of voice disorders in patients with FM is higher than that reported in normal subjects. The increased risk for voice disorders in patients with FM in comparison to healthy subjects can be attributed to involvement of the laryngeal muscles by FM. Like other skeletal muscles in the body, laryngeal muscles are subject to dysfunction as a result of decreased oxygenation and metabolic changes, although there are no electron microscopic studies assessing mitochondrial function in laryngeal muscles in FM patients. Similar to other skeletal muscles, laryngeal muscles rely on aerobic oxidative phosphorylation during normal speech. The voicing tasks used in daily communication usually are limited to phrases that last less than a minute. That said, the temporal constraint imposed by conversational requirements of speech and the low degree of force needed for conversation require limited muscle activity that relies mostly on aerobic metabolism. However, during intense voice tasks such as shouting and long performances, the laryngeal muscles may rely on anaerobic phosphorylation. The switch between the aerobic and anaerobic metabolic pathway depends mostly on the rigor of the voice task [39–42]. Impaired oxygenation of muscle tissue commonly described in FM also may be responsible for laryngeal muscle dysfunction and the increased risk for voice disorders in affected patients, although confirmatory studies have not been performed.

The speculations above extrapolated from our understanding of skeletal muscle pathophysiology in FM. Nevertheless, one must remain diligent regarding the disparity in muscle fiber composition between laryngeal and skeletal muscles. The muscle fiber composition of the intrinsic laryngeal muscles differs from that of limb muscles and varies markedly with the type of muscles, be it adductor, primarily phonatory vesus respiratory muscles, and with other functional characteristics. In a cadaver study, *Shiotani et al.* noted predominance of type IIa muscle fibers over type I and type IIb in all laryngeal muscles. There was a higher prevalence of type II fibers over type I fibers in the adductor muscles [39]. According to another cadaver study *by Li, et al*, fast type IIx fibers were present only in adductor muscles. The difference in muscle fiber type between laryngeal muscles and skeletal muscles has implications for muscle performance and type of metabolic pathway chosen by those muscle fibers. Slow-twitch type I fibers rely mostly on aerobic pathway to sustain low intense activity such as conversational speech, whereas type II fibers switch to anaerobic metabolism during fast and forceful contractions. Common examples include forceful and abrupt glottic closure to prevent aspiration and performance of high-intensity phonatory tasks [40, 41].

Another suggested explanation for the high prevalence of voice disorders in FM patients in comparison to controls is the proximity of the larynx to the cervical muscles. The high tension in the trapezius muscle in FM patients can spread easily to the adjacent strap muscles and to intrinsic laryngeal muscles resulting in tension and posing a risk for dysphonia. Another suggested mechanism is alteration in head position and pain-free mobility secondary to stiffness in the posterior muscles of the neck. Studies have shown that the use of ergonomically poor posture and/or exaggerated forward or backward head position may cause an increase in phonatory effort and thus predispose to dysphonia [43–45]. Patients with FM are known to suffer from high tension in the trapezius muscles which may lead to abnormal neck position. Similarly, deviation in posture due to low back pain or stiffness also many induce cervical muscle tension and alteration in laryngeal muscle function [46].

In addition, voice disorders in FM patient can be secondary to impairment in breathing, which is the main power source for phonation. The disturbances in breathing in FM are discussed thoroughly in Chap. 6 of this book.

In summary, the high prevalence of voice disorders in FM can be attributed to laryngeal dysfunction. Based on our understanding of the pathophysiology of skeletal muscle dysfunction in FM, it is fair to assume that laryngeal muscle dysfunction can be attributed to poor oxygenation, and to inflammatory and degenerative changes. Other possible causes include excess tension and asymmetry of the cervical muscles which can extend to the extrinsic and intrinsic laryngeal muscles leading to functional and possible structural voice disorders, and to changes in posture and respiration that can undermine support.

References

1. Jacobsen S, Danneskiold-Samsøe B. Isometric and isokinetic muscle strength in patients with fibrositis syndrome: new characteristics for a difficult definable category of patients. Scand J Rheumatol. 1987;16(1):61–5.
2. Mengshoel AM, Førre O, Komnaes HB. Muscle strength and aerobic capacity in primary fibromyalgia. Clin Exp Rheumatol. 1990;8(5):475–9.

3. Nordenskiöld UM, Grimby G. Grip force in patients with rheumatoid arthritis and fibromyalgia and in healthy subjects. A study with the Grippit instrument. Scand J Rheumatol. 1993;22(1):14–9.
4. Lindh MH, Göran L, Johansson A, Hedberg M, Grimby GL. Studies on maximal voluntary muscle contraction in patients with fibromyalgia. Arch Phys Med Rehabil. 1994;75(11):1217–22.
5. Nørregaard J, Bülow PM, Vestergaard-Poulsen P, Thomsen C, Danneskiold-Samøe B. Muscle strength, voluntary activation and cross-sectional muscle area in patients with fibromyalgia. Br J Rheumatol. 1995;34(10):925–31.
6. Nørregaard J, Bülow PM, Lykkegaard JJ, Mehlsen J, Danneskiold-Samsøoe B. Muscle strength, working capacity and effort in patients with fibromyalgia. Scand J Rehabil Med. 1997;29(2):97–102.
7. Maquet D, Croisier JL, Renard C, Crielaard JM. Muscle performance in patients with fibromyalgia. Joint Bone Spine. 2002;69(3):293–9.
8. Góes SM, Leite N, Shay BL, Homann D, Stefanello JM, Rodacki AL. Functional capacity, muscle strength and falls in women with fibromyalgia. Clin Biomech (Bristol). 2012;27(6):578–83.
9. Mülkoğlu C, Taşkın S, Vural S, Mansız Kaplan B, Selvi AB, Genç H. Isokinetic evaluation of the trunk muscle strength in housewives with fibromyalgia: a cross-sectional study. Adv Rheumatol. 2020;60(1):40.
10. Kapuczinski A, Soyfoo MS, De Breucker S, Margaux J. Assessment of sarcopenia in patients with fibromyalgia. Rheumatol Int. 2022;42(2):279–84.
11. Matthews PM, Allaire C, Shoubridge EA, Karpati G, Carpenter S, Arnold DL. In vivo muscle magnetic resonance spectroscopy in the clinical investigation of mitochondrial disease. Neurology. 1991;41(1):114–20.
12. Rubio-Zarapuz A, Parraca JA, Tornero-Aguilera JF, Clemente-Suárez VJ. Unveiling the link: exploring muscle oxygen saturation in fibromyalgia and its implications for symptomatology and therapeutic strategies. Med Gas Res. 2025;15(1):58–72.
13. Kalyan-Raman UP, Kalyan-Raman K, Yunus MB, Masi AT. Muscle pathology in primary fibromyalgia syndrome: a light microscopic, histochemical and ultrastructural study. J Rheumatol. 1984;11(6):808–13.
14. Lund N, Bengtsson A, Thorborg P. Muscle tissue oxygen pressure in primary fibromyalgia. Scand J Rheumatol. 1986;15(2):165–73.
15. Haljamäe H, Lewis DH, Hagberg H, Jennische E. Cellular effects of complete tourniquet ischemia. In: Induced skeletal muscle ischemia in man. Basil: Karger Publishers; 1982. p. 33–48.
16. Bengtsson A, Henriksson KG, Larsson J. Reduced high-energy phosphate levels in the painful muscles of patients with primary fibromyalgia. Arthritis Rheum. 1986;29(7):817–21.
17. Gerdle B, Ghafouri B, Lund E, Bengtsson A, Lundberg P, Ettinger-Veenstra HV, Leinhard OD, Forsgren MF. Evidence of mitochondrial dysfunction in fibromyalgia: deviating muscle energy metabolism detected using microdialysis and magnetic resonance. J Clin Med. 2020;9(11):3527. Electronic.
18. Villafaina S, Tomas-Carus P, Silva V, Costa AR, Fernandes O, Parraca JA. The behavior of muscle oxygen saturation, oxy and deoxy hemoglobin during a fatigue test in fibromyalgia. Biomedicines. 2023;11(1):132.
19. Inferrera F, Marino Y, D'Amico R, Impellizzeri D, Cordaro M, Siracusa R, Gugliandolo E, Fusco R, Cuzzocrea S, Di Paola R. Impaired mitochondrial quality control in fibromyalgia: mechanisms involved in skeletal muscle alteration. Arch Biochem Biophys. 2024;758:110083. Electronic.
20. Bengtsson A, Henriksson KG, Larsson J. Muscle biopsy in primary fibromyalgia. Light-microscopical and histochemical findings. Scand J Rheumatol. 1986;15(1):1–6.
21. Heffner RR, Barron SA. The early effects of ischemia upon skeletal muscle mitochondria. J Neurol Sci. 1978;38(3):295–315.
22. Umay E, Gundogdu I, Ozturk EA. What happens to muscles in fibromyalgia syndrome. Ir J Med Sci. 2020;189(2):749–56.

23. Wang H, Moser M, Schiltenwolf M, Buchner M. Circulating cytokine levels compared to pain in patients with fibromyalgia—a prospective longitudinal study over 6 months. J Rheumatol. 2008;35(7):1366–70.
24. Bennett RM. Beyond fibromyalgia: ideas on etiology and treatment. J Rheumatol Suppl. 1989;19:185–91.
25. Bennett RM, Clark SR, Goldberg L, Nelson D, Bonafede RP, Porter J, Specht D. Aerobic fitness in patients with fibrositis. A controlled study of respiratory gas exchange and 133xenon clearance from exercising muscle. Arthritis Rheum. 1989;32(4):454–60.
26. Jacobsen S, Petersen IS, Danneskiold-Samsøe B. Clinical features in patients with chronic muscle pain—with special reference to fibromyalgia. Scand J Rheumatol. 1993;22(2):69–76.
27. Vancampfort D, McGrath RL, Hemmings L, Gillis V, Bernar K, Van Damme T. Physical activity correlates in people with fibromyalgia: a systematic review. Disabil Rehabil. 2023;45(25):4165–74.
28. Vancampfort D, Brunner E, McGrath RL, Hemmings L, Van Damme T. Correlates of sedentary behavior in people with fibromyalgia: a systematic review. Int J Rheum Dis. 2023;26(5):841–9.
29. Karacay BC, Sahbaz T, Ceylan CM. The vicious cycle of physical inactivity, fatigue and kinesiophobia in patients with fibromyalgia syndrome. Reumatismo. 2022;74(4) https://doi.org/10.4081/reumatismo.2022.1502.
30. Gutiérrez L, Écija C, Catalá P, Peñacoba C. Sedentary behavior and pain after physical activity in women with fibromyalgia-the influence of pain-avoidance goals and catastrophizing. Biomedicines. 2023;11(1):154.
31. Werle E, Fisher H, Muller A, et al. Antibodies against serotonin have no diagnostic relevance in patients with fibromyalgia syndrome. J Rheumatol. 2001;28:595–600.
32. Greenfield S, Fitzcharles MA, Esdaile JM. Reactive fibromyalgia syndrome. Arthritis Rheum. 1992;1992(35):678–81.
33. Buskila D, Neumann L, Vaisberg G, Alkalay D, Wolfe F. ~~(1997)~~ Increased rates of fibromyalgia following cervical spine injury. A controlled study of 161 cases of traumatic injury. Arthritis Rheum. 1997;40:446–52.
34. Zetterman T, Markkula R, Partanen JV, Miettinen T, Estlander AM, Kalso E. Muscle activity and acute stress in fibromyalgia. BMC Musculoskelet Disord. 2021;22(1):183.
35. Cohen H, Buskila D, Neumann L, Ebstein RP. Confirmation of an association between fibromyalgia and serotonin transporter promoter region (5-HTTLPR) polymorphism, and relationship to anxiety-related personality traits. Arthritis Rheum. 2002;46(3):845–7.
36. Gursoy S, Erdal E, Herken H, Madenci E, Alasehirli B, Erdal N. Significance of catechol-O-methyltransferase gene polymorphism in fibromyalgia syndrome. Rheumatol Int. 2003;23:104–7.
37. Bueno-Antequera J, Munguía-Izquierdo D. Exercise and depressive disorder. Adv Exp Med Biol. 2020;1228:271–87.
38. Gavilán-Carrera B, Delgado-Fernández M, Sierra-Nieto E, et al. Sedentary time is associated with depressive symptoms and state anxiety in women with fibromyalgia. Could physical activity and fitness modify this association? The al-Ándalus project. Disabil Rehabil. 2023;45(20):3303–11.
39. Shiotani A, Westra WH, Flint PW. Myosin heavy chain composition in human laryngeal muscles. Laryngoscope. 1999;109(9):1521–4.
40. Li ZB, Lehar M, Nakagawa H, Foon Yoong Hoh J, Flint PW. Differential expression of myosin heavy chain isoforms between abductor and adductor muscles in the human larynx. Otolaryngol Head Neck Surg. 2004;130(2):217–22.
41. Morton-Jones ME, Gladden LB, Kavazis AN, Sandage MJ. A tutorial on skeletal muscle metabolism and the role of blood lactate: implications for speech production. J Speech Lang Hear Res. 2024;67(2):369–83.

42. Johnson AM, Sandage MJ. Exercise science and the vocalist. J Voice. 2021;35(4):668–77.
43. Gilman M, Johns MM. The effect of head position and/or stance on the self-perception of phonatory effort. J Voice. 2017;31(1):131.e1–4.
44. Rantala L, Sala E, Kankare E. Teachers' working postures and their effects on the voice. Folia Phoniatr Logop. 2018;70(1):24–36.
45. Franco D, Martins F, Andrea M, Fragoso I, Carrão L, Teles J. Is the sagittal postural alignment different in normal and dysphonic adult speakers? J Voice. 2014;28(4):523.e1–8.
46. Rubin JS, Blake E, Mathieson L, Kanana H. The effects of posture on voice. In: Sataloff RT. Professional voice. The science and art of clinical care. 4 San Diego: Plural Publishing; 2017. p. 1309–1318.

Autonomic Nervous System Dysfunction in Fibromyalgia and Its Effects on Voice

11

Abdul-latif Hamdan, Robert Thayer Sataloff, and Mary J. Hawkshaw

Autonomic Nervous System Dysfunction in Fibromyalgia (FM)

The autonomic nervous system (ANS) is responsible for control of homeostasis in the body. There is conflicting evidence about whether there is ANS dysfunction in Fibromyalgia (FM), and whether ANS dysfunction plays an etiologic role in this development or progression of the disease. Many studies have shown a higher prevalence of autonomic hyperfunction in FM patients, while others have shown no significant difference in comparison to healthy controls [1–6]. In 1992, *Yunus et al.* compared the plasma and serum levels of catecholamines in 30 patients with FM vs. 30 healthy controls and found no significant difference between the two groups. Moreover, there was no correlation between the clinical features of FM and levels of catecholamines [1]. However, *Lapossy et al.* detected a higher frequency of cold-induced vasospasm in patients with FM in comparison to controls and another group of patients with low back pain (38% vs. 8% vs. 20%, respectively). The degree of vasospasm, which was assessed using capillary hemodynamic blood flow analysis, correlated with pain intensity ($r = -0.383$). An increase in the degree of cold-induced vasospasm is considered a sign of heightened sympathetic activity suggestive of ANS dysfunction [2]. In 1988, *Bäckman et al.* assessed skeletal muscle function in patients with FM and noted lower maximum voluntary hand grip strength in comparison to controls. What was noticeable was the increase in the rate of muscle relaxation during sympathetic blockade in FM patients. The authors concluded that muscle dysfunction in FM is due to both central and peripheral etiologies [3]. In 1989, *Vaeroy et al.* examined the sympathetic nervous system in 27 patients with FM and found a lower vasoconstrictive response in comparison to 29 healthy controls. The authors used an auditory stimulus of 80 dB at 1000 Hz, and a hand cold pressor at 4 and 10 °C [4]. In 1997, *Boulaigah et al.* reported an abnormal sympathetic response to 45 min of 70° tilt in two thirds of patients with FM

A.-l. Hamdan et al., *Voice Disorders in Fibromyalgia*,
https://doi.org/10.1007/978-3-031-97751-0_11

compared to none in controls. There also was a differential increase in response between the study group and controls following isoproterenol infusion [5]. In 1998, *Martinez-Lavin et al.* investigated short-term heart rate variability in response to orthostatic stress in female atients with FM and noted derangement in the sympathetic response in comparison to healthy controls [6]. In 2014, Martinez-Martinez conducted a review exploring ANS dysfunction in chronic pain conditions including FM and noted predominance of the sympathetic nervous system in 65% of the studies examined. The authors discussed the role of ANS dysfunction in the pathogenesis of chronic pain symptoms [7]. In 2017, *Rizi et al.* investigated the influence of ANS dysfunction on sleep genesis in 50 FM patients and found an increase in heart rate and muscle sympathetic nerve activity at rest in comparison to controls, and a higher heart rate during sleep which correlated with the number of tender points. The authors deliberated on the vicious cycle of pain, heightened sympathetic activity and decrease in sleep efficacy in FM [8]. In 2020, *Del Paso* investigated sympathetic activity at rest in 45 FM patients using skin conductance as a measure of sweating. The results indicated a decrease in tonic skin conductance (SC) suggestive of reduced sympathetic activity. This was substantiated further by the lack of correlation between SC and state anxiety and body temperature [9].

There is growing evidence supporting sympathetic hyperactivity in patients with FM despite some reports indicating none. The sympathetic hyperactivity could be partially responsible for muscle dysfunction leading to muscle fatigue and decrease in strength. ANS dysfunction may also contribute to sleep disturbance in affected patients. More studies on the role of the ANS in FM are needed to elucidate the relationship.

Impact of ANS Dysfunction on Voice in FM Patients

There are no reports on the impact of ANS dysfunction on voice in FM patients. However, there are many reports on the link between the ANS and voice, particularly under stressful conditions such as performing highly demanding phonatory tasks. In 1989, *Orlikoff and Baken* conducted a study looking at the link between the cardiovascular system and fundamental frequency in 12 healthy subjects (6 males and 6 females). Patients were asked to sustain the vowel /ɑ/ at a comfortable pitch and loudness while the electrocardiographic (ECG) signal was recorded and monitored. Using signal averaging and autocorrelation, the authors found that the cardiovascular system accounted for 0.5%–20% of jitter, i.e., cycle-to-cycle variation in fundamental frequency. The influence of the cardiovascular system decreased with an increase in fundamental frequency [10]. In 2002, in a study that included 83 patients with non-organic habitual dysphonia, *Demmink-Geetman and Dejonckere* found that female patients had more ANS dysfunction than healthy controls. There was no correlation between the autonomic symptoms and dysphonia in men. The authors used the term "non-organic habitual dysphonia" in reference to patients with voice complaints and auditory perceptual deviance excluding those with structural lesions, spasmodic dysphonia, psychogenic dysphonia and/or hormone-induced changes [11]. In 2006, *Schneider et al.* investigated whether the increase in fundamental frequency after vocal loading was secondary to ANS dysfunction in 33 student teachers who had either a normal voice or "constitutional vocal hypofunction". A subject was classified as having a constitutionally weak voice if he or she could not reach a 90 DB SPL when asked to shout or sing loudly. Four autonomic parameters were recorded and measured at baseline and during a 1 h of teaching. These included heart rate, finger temperature, pulse transition time and voice fundamental frequency. The autonomic response was classified into four autonomic outlet types, autonomic outlet type 1 (AOT1) to AOT4, each denoting a different pattern of reaction to stress. The results showed no correlation between the increase in fundamental frequency and ANS reaction after 30 and 45 min of teaching [12]. In 2011, *Park and Behlau* investigated the symptoms and signs of ANS dysfunction in 61 patients with behavioral dysphonia in comparison to healthy controls with no voice complaints. Using a questionnaire that included questions related to "voice and autonomic nervous system", the authors showed a higher prevalence of neurovegetative symptoms and signs in patients with dysphonia in comparison to those with no dysphonia. The most common symptoms were the need for repetitive swallowing, throat clearing, sore throat and voice fatigue [13]. In 2013, *Alvear et al.* investigated the influence of heart rate variability on fundamental frequency while subjects were asked to perform three classic autonomic tasks, namely the isometric hand grip, the mental arithmetic task and the cutaneous cold test. The authors noted a significant association between cardiovascular changes and voice frequency [14]. In 2014, *Helou et al.* examined the impact of ANS activation on intrinsic laryngeal muscle activity in eight healthy volunteers. Activation of the ANS was achieved using cold compressors, and intrinsic laryngeal muscle activity was measured using electromyography. The results showed a parallel increase in adductor and abductor muscles activity with the increase in heart rate and blood pressure. The authors highlighted the link between intrinsic laryngeal msucle activity and stress [15]. During same year, *Cunha et al.* reported the link between the Voice Handicap Index (VHI) score and heart rate variability in physical education teachers. The results showed a correlation between the functional and organic domains of the VHI and the high frequency index of heart rate variability. The authors concluded that autonomic regulation had an effect on voice [16]. In 2017, *MacPherson et al.* investigated the impact of increased cognitive load on 4 acoustic variables and 3 measures of autonomic arousal, namely pulse period and volume amplitude, and skin conductance. While 16 healthy volunteers were asked to read a sentence with two load conditions, acoustic and autonomic measures were recorded. The results showed an association between cognitive load, low-to-high spectral energy and cepstral peak prominence [17].

In summary, there are no studies on the impact of ANS dysfunction on voice in FM patients but there are many studies documenting the strong link between the ANS and voice, and on the link between FM and ANS An increase in sympathetic activity can result in an increase in the activity of the intrinsic laryngeal muscles and alteration in some of the acoustic parameters. Similarly, patients with behavioral dysphonia are more likely to experience neuro-vegetative symptoms suggestive of autonomic nervous system dysfunction. Future investigations on the effect of ANS on voice in FM patients are needed.

References

1. Yunus MB, Dailey JW, Aldag JC, Masi AT, Jobe PC. Plasma and urinary catecholamines in primary fibromyalgia: a controlled study. J Rheumatol. 1992;19(1):95–7.
2. Lapossy E, Gasser P, Hrycaj P, Dubler B, Samborski W, Muller W. Cold-induced vasospasm in patients with fibromyalgia and chronic low back pain in comparison to healthy subjects. Clin Rheumatol. 1994;13(3):442–5.
3. Bäckman E, Bengtsson A, Bengtsson M, Lennmarken C, Henriksson KG. Skeletal muscle function in primary fibromyalgia. Effect of regional sympathetic blockade with guanethidine. Acta Neurol Scand. 1988;77(3):187–91.
4. Vaerøy H, Qiao ZG, Mørkrid L, Førre O. Altered sympathetic nervous system response in patients with fibromyalgia (fibrositis syndrome). J Rheumatol. 1989;16(11):1460–5.
5. Bou-Holaigah I, Calkins H, Flynn JA, Tunin C, Chang HC, Kan JS, Rowe PC. Provocation of hypotension and pain during upright tilt table testing in adults with fibromyalgia. Clin Exp Rheumatol. 1997;15(3):239–46.
6. Martínez-Lavín M, Hermosillo AG, Rosas M, Soto ME. Circadian studies of autonomic nervous balance in patients with fibromyalgia: a heart rate variability analysis. Arthritis Rheum. 1998;41(11):1966–71.
7. Martínez-Martínez LA, Mora T, Vargas A, Fuentes-Iniestra M, Martínez-Lavín M. Sympathetic nervous system dysfunction in fibromyalgia, chronic fatigue syndrome, irritable bowel syndrome, and interstitial cystitis: a review of case-control studies. J Clin Rheumatol. 2014;20(3):146–50.
8. Rizzi M, Radovanovic D, Santus P, Airoldi A, Frassanito F, Vanni S, Cristiano A, Masala IF, Sarzi-Puttini P. Influence of autonomic nervous system dysfunction in the genesis of sleep disorders in fibromyalgia patients. Clin Exp Rheumatol. 2017;35 Suppl 105(3):74–80.
9. Reyes Del Paso GA, de la Coba P. Reduced activity, reactivity and functionality of the sympathetic nervous system in fibromyalgia: an electrodermal study. PLoS One. 2020;15(10):e0241154.
10. Orlikoff RF, Baken RJ. The effect of the heartbeat on vocal fundamental frequency perturbation. J Speech Hear Res. 1989;32(3):576–82.
11. Demmink-Geertman L, Dejonckere PH. Nonorganic habitual dysphonia and autonomic dysfunction. J Voice. 2002;16(4):549–59.
12. Schneider B, Enne R, Cecon M, Diendorfer-Radner G, Wittels P, Bigenzahn W, Johannes B. Effects of vocal constitution and autonomic stress-related reactivity on vocal endurance in female student teachers. J Voice. 2006;20(2):242–50.
13. Park K, Behlau M. Sinais e sintomas da disfunção autônoma em indivíduos disfônicos [Signs and symptoms of autonomic dysfunction in dysphonic individuals]. J Soc Bras Fonoaudiol. 2011;23(2):164–9. Portuguese.
14. Alvear RM, Barón-López FJ, Alguacil MD, Dawid-Milner MS. Interactions between voice fundamental frequency and cardiovascular parameters. Preliminary results and physiological mechanisms. Logoped Phoniatr Vocol. 2013;38(2):52–8.

15. Helou LB, Wang W, Ashmore RC, Rosen CA, Abbott KV. Intrinsic laryngeal muscle activity in response to autonomic nervous system activation. Laryngoscope. 2013;123(11):2756–65.
16. Cunha DS, de Abreu LC, Frizzo AC, Cardoso MA, Valenti VE. Vocal complaint in physical education teachers and its association with the cardiovascular system. Int Arch Med. 2014;7(1):7.
17. MacPherson MK, Abur D, Stepp CE. Acoustic measures of voice and physiologic measures of autonomic arousal during speech as a function of cognitive load. J Voice. 2017;31(4):504.e1–9.

The Effect on Voice of Sleep Disorders in Fibromyalgia

12

Abdul-latif Hamdan, Robert Thayer Sataloff, and Mary J. Hawkshaw

The Link Between Sleep Disorders and Fibromyalgia

The symptoms of Fibromyalgia (FM) are not limited to the musculoskeletal system. Affected patients present with a numerous of extra-skeletal complaints including is impairment in sleep. There is growing evidence in the literature supporting a bi-directional relationship between sleep disorders and FM [1, 2]. *Theadom et al.* explored sleep disorders in 101 patients diagnosed with FM and reported poor sleep quality in 99% of their participants [1]. *Biagtti et al.* investigated 600 patients with FM and noted sleep disturbance in 96% of their study group. The sleep disturbance persisted in 94.7% of those who were followed for 1 year (n = 492) [2]. *Ughreja et al.* investigated the sleep of 86 patients with FM using validated questionnaires and found that 91% were poor sleepers. There was a moderate positive correlation between the Pittsburgh Sleep Quality Index score [3] and the FM Impact Questionnaire score ($r = 0.4$) [4]. Poor sleep quality led to worsening of pain and the psychological state of affected patients [5]. *Singh et al.* conducted a cross-sectional study on 100 FM patients and noted a correlation between pain severity and sleep quality. Patient with severe FM had worse sleep quality compared to those with less severe FM. The poor sleep quality also correlated with anxiety and depression [6]. In another study on 20 patients with FM, *Cervilla et al.* reported subjective sleep disturbance in all the participants. The disturbance in sleep quality was associated with the severity of pain and with depression. The authors highlighted the need to address mental comorbidities in FM patients with sleep disorders [7]. Sleep disturbances also have been shown to be a risk factor for FM. Using a survey on gender-specific differences in patients with OSA, *Wahner-Roedler et al.* noted that women with obstructive sleep apnea (OSA) were more likely to have FM and irritable bowel syndrome among other comorbidities which included obesity and depression [8]. In a systematic review by *He et al*, the authors reported that the collective incidence of FM in patients with OSA is 21% [9].

A.-l. Hamdan et al., *Voice Disorders in Fibromyalgia*,
https://doi.org/10.1007/978-3-031-97751-0_12

Several types of sleep alterations have been described in FM, the most common of which is the "non-restorative sleep". In 1975, *Moldofsky et al.* suggested the term "non-restorative sleep syndrome" in reference to symptoms such as delay in onset of sleep, poor sleep quality and non-freshening sleep. The term "alpha-delta" sleep was introduced to describe the presence of alpha-delta waves on electro-encephalogram (EEG) during non-rapid eye movement (NREM) sleep, which is thought to be responsible for non-freshening sleep [10]. *Branco et al.* examined the alpha and delta activity during a night-long sleep in ten patients with FM and noted the occurrence of alpha-delta patterns in almost all the participants. In addition to the high prevalence of alpha electro-encephalogram (EEG) NREM sleep, most patients had increase in awakening and sleep fragmentation [11]. *Roizenblatt et al.* investigated the alpha sleep activity in NREM sleep in 40 female patients with FM and found different patterns in comparison to healthy controls. There was a correlation between the clinical manifestations of FM in terms of pain and tender points and the phasic alpha sleep activity pattern [12]. These findings were in accord with a study by *Moldofsky et al.* that investigated the impact of stage four selective sleep stage deprivation on musculoskeletal pain in six patients with FM [13]. The authors found an increase in musculoskeletal symptoms and in musculoskeletal tenderness in comparison to baseline. The authors speculated on the association between NREM sleep and FM symptoms [13]. Similarly, in a study that included 101 FM patients, *Theadom et al.* noted that poor sleep quality significantly predicted fatigue and pain. The authors suggested the need to improve sleep quality in order to better the overall quality of life of FM patients [1].

The pathogenesis of non-restorative sleep in patients with FM is complex. One hypothesis is disturbance in the hypothalamic-pituitary axis (HPA) resulting in alteration in cortisol response and other hormonal responses that may be responsible for sleep disturbance and chronic fatigue [14–16]. Another suggested mechanism is hyperactivity of the sympathetic nervous system with subsequent increase in heart rate variability [17, 18]. In a study on sympathetic nervous system function in 13 female patients with FM, *Torpy et al.* reported higher baseline norepinephrine levels in FM patients compared to controls. Moreover, the increase in the norepinephrine level 1–3 h after the administration of interleukin-6 (IL-6) was higher in patients with FM in comparison to a control group matched by age, gender and body mass index. The exaggerated response, i.e., increase in norepinephrine release, and the delay in adeno-corticotropic hormone (ACTH) release following IL-6 administration suggested dysregulation in the sympathetic nervous system [15]. Other suggested mechanisms for the non-restorative sleep include the release of pro-inflammatory cytokines, physical or psychological distress and genetic predisposition [18, 19].

Another sleep disorder that has been discussed thoroughly in the context of FM is OSA. There are numerous studies indicating that FM increases the risk of OSA. *Jennum* et al. evaluated the sleep of 40 patients with FM and noted a higher percent arousal time and index in comparison to controls. Polysomnography conducted on 20 of those patients revealed an apnea/hypopnea index above 5 in 50% of the cases versus in only two out of ten controls. Using a self-reported questionnaire, the authors also showed higher prevalence of insomnia, daytime fatigability and cognitive disturbance which could have been attributed to sleep fragmentation [20]. *May et al.* conducted polysomnography on FM patients (n = 117, 92 women and 25 men) suspected of having sleep disorders and found that 44% of the male participants had evidence of sleep apnea. The patient was considered to have sleep apnea if he had at least five apnea-hypopnea events per hour with duration of each exceeding 10 s. The authors noted also that FM could be a clinical index for non-diagnosed or subclinical sleep apnea in men [21]. *Sergi et al.* investigated the sleep of 17 patients with FM using polysomnography and noted that affected patients slept less efficiently than healthy controls, had more arousals, and had a higher number of oxygen desaturations per hour of sleep. With respect to the pattern of breathing, 15 of 17 had high periodic breathing in comparison to only 2 out of 17 controls. In addition, those who complained of daytime hypersomnolence had a higher number of tender points on examination [22]. *Cetin et al.* investigated sleep quality in 33 patients with FM using polysomnography and noted that 12 had OSA. The high Pittsburgh Sleep Quality index [3] and the Epworth Sleepiness Scale scores [23] also indicated that FM patients had poorer sleep quality associated with a significantly higher number of arousals and awakenings in comparison to controls. The authors stressed the need to evaluate FM patients with sleep alteration for the presence of OSA [24]. *Mutlu et al.* examined the prevalence of OSA in 38 patients with FM and found that almost two thirds had OSA. There was a moderate negative correlation between the AHI score and the physical functioning subscale of the 36-item short form Health survey (SF-36) [25] (p less than 0.001). Moreover, there was a positive correlation between disease-activity score and the Apnea-hypopnea index [26].

Another less frequently described sleep-related disorder in patients with FM is Upper Airway Resistance Syndrome (UARS). Upper airway resistance syndrome is a form of sleep disorder characterized by increased collapsibility of the upper airway, the extent of which is intermediate between normal and mild-to-moderate OSA [27, 28]. *Gold et al.* investigated the prevalence of UARS in 28 women with FM in comparison to 11 women diagnosed with UARS and noted comparable results between the two groups in regard to inspiratory flow limitation, arousal index and AHI. Only one patient was diagnosed with obstructive sleep apnea-hypopnea while 26 of the 28 had inspiratory airflow limitation with arousals. In view of the high prevalence of inspiratory airflow limitation in their study group (96%), and given that UARS is a common cause of fatigue and daytime sleepiness secondary to sleep fragmentation, the authors suggested the possible pathogenic role of UARS in the development of some of the somatic complaints reported in FMS [29].

The higher prevalence of OSA and UARS in Fibromyalgia can be ascribed to the high BMI in some affected patients. Obesity is a common comorbidity in FM affecting a very high percentage of patients. The main causes include reduced activity, sedentary behavior and alteration in the neuroendocrine system. A thorough discussion on the pathogenesis of obesity in FM is available to readers in Chap. 14 of this book.

The prevalence of sleep impairment in FM is very high. The most commonly reported sleep disorders are "non-restorative sleep", OSA and UARS. The pathophysiology of sleep disorders in FM is complex. Suggested mechanisms include disturbance in the HPA, hyperactivity of the sympathetic nervous system, metabolic disorders and mechanical factors such as narrowing of the upper airway. Sleep disturbances are associated with daytime fatigability and impaired cognitive function. Hence, when present, sleep disturbances may exacerbate the symptoms of FM and lead to worse quality of life. Patients with FM and refractory symptoms need to be assessed for the presence of sleep disorders.

The Impact of Sleep Disorders on Voice in FM Patients

There are no studies on the impact of sleep deprivation on voice in FM patients. However, there are numerous reports on the link between sleep and voice. Sleep deprivation is known to affect various systems in the body including the phonatory system. *Cho et al.* conducted a cross-sectional study looking at the correlation between subjective voice problems and duration of sleep and noted that sleeping less than 5 h or more than 9 h increased the risk of hoarseness. The odds ratio were 1.45 and 1.365, respectively. The impact of sleep deprivation or excess sleep on voice was seen more in men compared to women [30]. *Hong et al.* investigated the association between OSA and benign lesions of the vocal folds and found that OSA increased the risk of developing benign lesion by 79% in comparison to controls. The risk increased with age and female gender [31]. *Thoret et al.* investigated the effect of sleep deprivation on voice using automated acoustic analysis and showed the presence of temporal changes of prosody in addition to alteration in spectral features. The authors stressed the individual variations and highlighted the utility of voice biomarkers in detecting sleep deprivation. The term "sleep stethoscopes" was introduced as a new diagnostic tool for sleep deprivation [32]. *Icht et al.* performed acoustic analysis on 47 participants following nocturnal sleep and sleep deprivation for 24 h. The results showed an increase in harmonic-to-noise ratio after sleep deprivation, meaning that the voice quality had more periodic sounds compared to noise (aperiodic) hence clearer voice in patients who had been awake for 24 h than in those who had slept. The effect was more seen in female participants compared to male participants. The authors attributed these changes to asynchronous vocal fold vibration following sleep, changes in the distribution of fluids in the mucous membranes of the throat region that occur during nocturnal sleep, dryness of the vocal folds due to mouth breathing, and gastric reflux during sleep [33]. The term "flattening" of the voice in reference to loss of intonation has also been described particularly in Professional voice users who are extremely vulnerable to sleep-induced physiologic changes. When challenged with sleep deprivation in addition to the stress of performance, voice quality is in jeopardy [34].

Sleep deprivation is known to reduce functional capacity and increase work-related injuries. It is a major cause of neurocognitive changes and mood alteration which can impact our means of communication. The impact of sleep deprivation on voice is not understood thoroughly and several theories have been suggested. These include dysfunction in fine neuromuscular control of vocal fold condition and motion, alteration in inflammatory response and immunologic-induced changes [35]. Another possible explanation is obesity. Numerous reports indicate that FM patients with sleep disorders are more likely to have a high BMI in comparison to healthy controls, and that obesity per se is a risk factor for dysphonia [36–39]. In a study on the relationship between obesity and FM, Okifuji et al. reported a negative correlation between body mass index (BMI), sleep efficiency and total sleep time ($r = -0.44$ and $r = -0.56$, respectively). The authors highlighted the adverse role of obesity in Fibromyalgia-related dysfunction [40]. With an increase in BMI, obese patients with sleep disorders are more likely to be mouth breather. Mouth breathing and snoring can lead to laryngeal desiccation and predispose to voice disorders. More information on this topic is available to the readers in the book "Obesity and Voice" [41].

There are no studies on the link between sleep disturbances and dysphonia in FM patients. However, the adverse effect of sleep disorders on voice in FM patients can be extrapolated from our understanding of the pathophysiology of dysphonia in patients with impairment in sleep, and the clear association between FM and sleep disturbance. Suggested mechanisms include sleep-induced autonomic nervous system dysfunction and obesity-related changes which may jeopardize all three components of the vocal apparatus. Future research on the association between sleep and voice disorders in FM is needed.

References

1. Theadom A, Cropley M, Humphrey KL. Exploring the role of sleep and coping in quality of life in fibromyalgia. J Psychosom Res. 2007;62:145–51.
2. Bigatti SM, Hernandez AM, Cronan TA, Rand KL. Sleep disturbances in fibromyalgia syndrome: relationship to pain and depression. Arthritis Rheum. 2008;59:961–7.
3. Buysse DJ, Reynolds CF III, Monk TH, Berman SR, Kupfer DJ. The pittsburgh sleep quality index: a new instrument for psychiatric practice and research. Psychiatry Res. 1989;28:193–213.
4. Burckhardt CS, Clark S, Bennett RM. The fibromyalgia impact questionnaire: development and validation. J Rheumatol. 1991;18:728–33.
5. Ughreja RA, Venkatesan P, Gopalakrishna DB, Singh YP, Vani Lakshmi R. Sleep profile and its correlation with clinical variables in fibromyalgia syndrome: a cross-sectional study. J Taibah Univ Med Sci. 2023;19(1):90–8.
6. Singh R, Rai NK, Pathak A, Rai J, Pakhare A, Kashyap PV, Rozatkar AR, Mishra S, Mudda S. Impact of fibromyalgia severity on patients mood, sleep quality, and quality of life. J Neurosci Rural Pract. 2024;15(2):320–6.
7. Cervilla O, Miró E, Martínez MP, Sánchez AI, Sabio JM, Prados G. Sleep quality and clinical and psychological manifestations in women with mild systemic lupus erythematosus activity compared to women with fibromyalgia: a preliminary study. Mod Rheumatol. 2020;30(6):1016–24.

8. Wahner-Roedler DL, Olson EJ, Narayanan S, Sood R, Hanson AC, Loehrer LL, Sood A. Gender-specific differences in a patient population with obstructive sleep apnea-hypopnea syndrome. Gend Med. 2007;4(4):329–38.
9. He J, Chen M, Huang N, Wang B. Fibromyalgia in obstructive sleep apnea-hypopnea syndrome: a systematic review and meta-analysis. Front Physiol. 2024;15:1394865.
10. Moldofsky H, Scarisbrick P, England R, Smythe H. Musculosketal symptoms and non-REM sleep disturbance in patients with "fibrositis syndrome" and healthy subjects. Psychosom Med. 1975;37(4):341–51.
11. Branco J, Atalaia A, Paiva T. Sleep cycles and alpha-delta sleep in fibromyalgia syndrome. J Rheumatol. 1994;21(6):1113–7.
12. Roizenblatt S, Moldofsky H, Benedito-Silva AA, Tufik S. Alpha sleep characteristics in fibromyalgia. Arthritis Rheum. 2001;44(1):222–30.
13. Moldofsky H, Scarisbrick P. Induction of neurasthenic musculoskeletal pain syndrome by selective sleep stage deprivation. Psychosom Med. 1976;38(1):35–44.
14. Adler GK, Manfredsdottir VF, Creskoff KW. Neuroendocrine abnormalities in fibromyalgia. Curr Pain Headache Rep. 2002;6:289–98.
15. Torpy DJ, Papanicolaou DA, Lotsikas AJ, Wilder RL, Chrousos GP, Pillemer SR. Responses of the sympathetic nervous system and the hypothalamic-pituitary-adrenal axis to interleukin-6: a pilot study in fibromyalgia. Arthritis Rheum. 2000;43:872–80.
16. Calis M, Gokce C, Ates F, Ulker S, Izgi HB, Demir H, et al. Investigation of the hypothalamo-pituitary-adrenal axis (HPA) by 1 microg ACTH test and metyrapone test in patients with primary fibromyalgia syndrome. J Endocrinol Investig. 2004;27:42–6.
17. Chervin RD, Teodorescu M, Kushwaha R, Deline AM, Brucksch CB, Ribbens-Grimm C, et al. Objective measures of disordered sleep in fibromyalgia. J Rheumatol. 2009;36:2009–16.
18. Martinez-Lavin M, Hermosillo AG. Autonomic nervous system dysfunction may explain the multisystem features of fibromyalgia. Semin Arthritis Rheum. 2000;29:197–9.
19. Abeles AM, Pillinger MH, Solitar BM, Abeles M. Narrative review: the pathophysiology of fibromyalgia. Ann Intern Med. 2007;146:726–34.
20. Jennum P, Drewes AM, Andreasen A, Nielsen KD. Sleep and other symptoms in primary fibromyalgia and in healthy controls. J Rheumatol. 1993;20(10):1756–9.
21. May KP, West SG, Baker MR, Everett DW. Sleep apnea in male patients with the fibromyalgia syndrome. Am J Med. 1993;94(5):505–8.
22. Sergi M, Rizzi M, Braghiroli A, Sarzi Puttini P, Greco M, Cazzola M, Andreoli A. Periodic breathing during sleep in patients affected by fibromyalgia syndrome. Eur Respir J. 1999;14(1):203–8.
23. Johns MW. A new method for measuring daytime sleepiness: the Epworth sleepiness scale. Sleep. 1991;14(6):540–5.
24. Çetin B, Sünbül EA, Toktaş H, Karaca M, Ulutaş Ö, Güleç H. Comparison of sleep structure in patients with fibromyalgia and healthy controls. Sleep Breath. 2020;24(4):1591–8.
25. Koçyiğit H, Aydemir Ö, Fisek G, Ölmez N, Memiş A. Reliability and validity of the Turkish version of short-form-36 (SF-36). İlaçve Tedavi Dergisi. 1999;12:102–6.
26. Mutlu P, Zateri C, Zohra A, Ozerdogan O, Mirici AN. Prevalence of obstructive sleep apnea in female patients with fibromyalgia. Saudi Med J. 2020;41(7):740–5.
27. Gold AR, Marcus CL, Dipalo F, Gold MS. Upper airway collapsibility during sleep in upper airway resistance syndrome. Chest. 2002;121(5):1531–40.
28. Guilleminault C, Stoohs R, Clerk A, Cetel M, Maistros P. A cause of excessive daytime sleepiness. The upper airway resistance syndrome. Chest. 1993;104(3):781–7.
29. Gold AR, Dipalo F, Gold MS, Broderick J. Inspiratory airflow dynamics during sleep in women with fibromyalgia. Sleep. 2004;27(3):459–66.
30. Cho JH, Guilminault C, Joo YH, Jin SK, Han KD, Park CS. A possible association between dysphonia and sleep duration: a cross-sectional study based on the Korean National Health and nutrition examination surveys from 2010 to 2012. PLoS One. 2017;12(8):e0182286.

31. Hong YT, Kang MG, Lee MG, Yeom SW, Kim JS. Association between obstructive sleep apnea and risk of benign vocal fold lesions: a nationwide 9-year follow-up cohort study. Medicine (Baltimore). 2024;103(25):e38447.
32. Thoret E, Andrillon T, Gauriau C, Léger D, Pressnitzer D. Sleep deprivation detected by voice analysis. PLoS Comput Biol. 2024;20(2):e1011849.
33. Icht M, Zukerman G, Hershkovich S, Laor T, Heled Y, Fink N, Fostick L. The "morning voice": the effect of 24–hours of sleep deprivation on vocal parameters of young adults. J Voice. 2020;34(3):489.e1–9.
34. Sataloff RT. Professional voice: the science and art of clinical care. San Diego: Plural Publishing; 2017.
35. Rocha BR, Behlau M. The influence of sleep disorders on voice quality. J Voice. 2018;32(6):771.e1–771.e13.
36. Yunus MB, Arslan S, Aldag JC. Relationship between body mass index and fibromyalgia features. Scand J Rheumatol. 2002;31(1):27–31.
37. Aparicio VA, Ortega FB, Carbonell-Baeza A, Camiletti D, Ruiz JR, Delgado-Fernández M. Relationship of weight status with mental and physical health in female fibromyalgia patients. Obes Facts. 2011;4(6):443–8.
38. Kim CH, Luedtke CA, Vincent A, Thompson JM, Oh TH. Association of body mass index with symptom severity and quality of life in patients with fibromyalgia. Arthritis Care Res (Hoboken). 2012;64(2):222–8.
39. Atzeni F, Alciati A, Salaffi F, et al. The association between body mass index and fibromyalgia severity: data from a cross-sectional survey of 2339 patients. Rheumatol Adv Pract. 2021;5(1):rkab015.
40. Okifuji A, Bradshaw DH, Olson C. Evaluating obesity in fibromyalgia: neuroendocrine biomarkers, symptoms, and functions. Clin Rheumatol. 2009;28(4):475–8.
41. Hamdan AL, Sataloff RT, Hawkshaw MJ. Obesity and voice. San Diego: Plural Publishing; 2019.

Chronic Fatigue Syndrome, Depression, Fibromyalgia and Voice

13

Abdul-latif Hamdan, Robert Thayer Sataloff,
and Mary J. Hawkshaw

Chronic Fatigue Syndrome, Fibromyalgia and Voice

Chronic Fatigue Syndrome in Fibromyalgia

Chronic fatigue syndrome (CFS) is a condition characterized by chronic idiopathic fatigue and pain. The pain is not limited to muscles but involves joints, throat and lymph nodes in various areas in the body [1, 2]. Associated symptoms include decrease in cognitive ability, sleep disturbance, headache, and mood alteration. Over two million Americans and close to 3% of the world population are affected by this syndrome [3]. Patients are usually in their fifth and sixth decades of life, with a higher prevalence being noted in women compared to men [4]. In many instances, the onset of symptoms follows an upper respiratory tract infection which is why CFS has been associated with viral infections most common of which is Epstein virus (EBV) [5].

Chronic fatigue syndrome is a disabling disorder that worsens the quality of life at many fronts. The extent of functional impairment can lead to a decrease in productivity and absenteeism. In a survey that included 298 patients with CFS, *Vercoulen et al.* identified nine dimensions of impairment in the life of affected subjects. These included self-efficacy, psychological well-being and social functioning in addition to other sleep and daily- related activities. The authors stressed the need for a multidimensional approach in the assessment and treatment of patients [6]. The diagnosis of CFS is hard to make given the complexity of this syndrome. Several diagnostic criteria have been set most important of which are the ones described by the Center for Disease Control and Prevention in 1988, and later revised in 1994 [7]. Other adopted criteria are the Oxford criteria described in 1991 [8]. These criteria are being revisited

A.-l. Hamdan et al., *Voice Disorders in Fibromyalgia*,
https://doi.org/10.1007/978-3-031-97751-0_13

frequently to further emphasize the mental fatigue and disability over the physical symptoms. The work-up of suspected CFS patients should be comprehensive and focused on excluding other causes of muscle and joint pain. Any pathology indicative of a structural disorder, neurologic or psychologic disability should be ruled out. In addition to a thorough history taking and physical examination, a full battery of blood tests should be performed including auto-antibody screens, viral titers in addition to the basic complete blood count, chemistry analysis and thyroid function testing.

There is a major overlap in the demographic characteristics and clinical presentation of patients with CFS and Fibromyalgia (FM) making the distinction between these two disorders a challenging task. In both syndromes, women are more affected than men, and patients present with diffuse body aches, long-lasting fatigue, decrease in work tolerance, cognitive impairment, sleep disturbances and insomnia [9]. Other common co-morbidities include neural- mediated hypotension and dysregulation in growth-hormone-insulin-like growth factor [10]. The similarity in the clinical presentation of patients with CFS and FM has fueled investigations looking for a common pathophysiology, most important of which is central sensitization. *Bourke et al.* investigated central sensitization in 19 patients with FM and 19 cases of CFS in comparison to 20 healthy controls. The authors found reduced pain threshold in CFS and FM cases compared to healthy controls. Moreover, patients with FM had decreased cold-induced pain threshold and increased heat-induced pain threshold in comparison to controls. The overall prevalence of central sensitization in FM cases and CFS cases was 95% and 84%, respectively. The authors concluded that central sensitization may be a common pathophysiology for both syndromes [11]. Other suggested shared pathophysiologic mechanisms aside from central sensitization include alteration in the immune system, dysfunction neuroendocrine system, and genetic predisposition [5, 12–16],

The link between CFS and FM remains very complex despite the advances in diagnostic and therapeutic methods. The clinical presentation between the two conditions overlaps in various domains suggesting a common pathophysiology, namely central sensitization. Physicians should be diligent in the work-up and treatment of patients presenting with diffuse body pain and fatigue.

Impact of CFS on Voice in FM Patients

There are no studies in the literature on voice disorders in FM patients with CFS, however it is well established that CFS increases the risk of voice disorders. This is understandable given that CFS is a musculoskeletal disorder and that the laryngeal muscles are skeletal muscles similar to other muscles in the body. *Piersiala et al.* investigated the laryngeal manifestations of 215 patients with chronic pain syndromes, 70 of whom with CFS, and noted an increase in the odds of having functional voice disorders in comparison to a control group (OR 1.525, CI 0.956). The authors concluded that CFS, among other chronic pain syndromes, is a risk factor for functional voice disorders [17]. Chronic fatigue syndrome may also affect voice secondary to associated comorbidities such as sleep disturbance and autonomic nervous system dysfunction. Sleep deprivation can lead to voice fatigue [18–20], and dysfunction in the autonomic nervous system may lead to alteration in many acoustic variables [21–23]. Similarly, impairment in cognitive capacity which is commonly reported in CFS may jeopardize voice particularly in professional voice users [24],

There are no studies in the literature on the impact of CFS on voice in FM patients. However, many studies indicate that patients with CFS are at a higher risk of developing functional voice disorders in comparison to healthy individuals. The effect of CFS on voice may be direct or secondary to associated comorbidities. Future research on voice disorders in FM patients with CFS is warranted.

Depression, Fibromyalgia and Voice

Depression in Fibromyalgia

Fibromyalgia is a chronic disabling condition of unknown etiology. It is a polymorphic syndrome associated with a heterogenous number of systemic disturbances including the neuropsychic system. Patients with FM often display explicit personality traits such perfectionism, obsessive-compulsiveness, high-self transcendence, and low-self-esteem. What is alarming is the high prevalence of psychiatric comorbidities in association with these personality traits. Numerous studies showed a high prevalence of anxiety, depression, and post-traumatic stress disorders in FM patients, the impact of which on quality of life is significant [25, 26]. Using a structured clinical interview for the assessment of mental disorders in a cohort of 115 patients with FM, *Thieme et al.* noted a difference in the prevalence of anxiety in relation to the psychosocial traits of affected patients. Anxiety disorder was reported in 67.7% of patients in the dysfunctional group in comparison to 15% in the interpersonally distress group and 19.5% in the adaptive copers group. On the other hand, depression was more prevalent in the interpersonally distressed group in comparison to the other two groups. The authors stressed the need to address both the emotional and physical burden of the disease [27]. *Fietta et al.* reviewed the link between FM and psychiatric disorders and noted the prevalence of anxiety and depression in 13–63.8% and 20–80% of the cases, respectively [28]. In a survey that included 350 FM patients, *AlZabibi* et al. noted major depressive disorder as a significant risk factor that increased the odds of being diagnosed with FM (OR = 2.62, CI 95%). Other factors included irritable bowel syndrome and restless leg syndrome [29]. In another cross-sectional study, *Sadr et al.* reported the prevalence of at least one psychiatric disorder in 92% of patients with FM, and the prevalence of anxiety disorders in 16.98% of the cases. Their cohort consisted of 159 patients and psychiatric assessment was made via interviews over the course of 2 years [30]. *Gardoki-Souto et al.* examined the prevalence of psychological trauma in 88 female patients with FM and noted history of a major traumatic event in 84% of the cases. Moreover,

71.5% of the participants had met the diagnostic criteria of PTSD, and all patients exhibited symptoms of anxiety and depression in various levels. The level of pain was predictive of mental disorders and poor quality of life [31]. In a systematic review on the impact of treating major depressive disorder in patients with various medical illnesses including FM, *Arnaud et al.* noted significant reduction of chronic pain following treatment. Improvement in depressive symptoms led to an improvement on many medical conditions among which is Fibromyalgia [32].

There is no clear understanding why the high prevalence of mental illnesses in FM patients. One suggested hypothesis is the increase in body weight [33]. *Aparicio et al.* examined the association between weight, anxiety and depression in a cohort of female patients with FM and noted that normal-weight patients had less anxiety and depression than obese patients. There was no statistical difference in the levels of anxiety and depression between overweight and obese patients. The mental health score using the SF-36 was worse in the overweight and obese subgroups which accounted for 35% and 33% of the total group, respectively [33]. These findings are not surprising given the higher prevalence of psychiatric disorders in obese subjects in comparison to normal weight subjects. In a study on obesity and the impact of chronic pain, *Marcus et al.* noted that obese patients had higher beck Depression Inventory score (15.78 ± 9.88 in comparison to overweight or normal weight patients (12.88 ± 11.64 and 11.81 ± 7.55, respectively) [34]. *Kelly et al.* evaluated the link between obesity, distress and suicidal ideation in a large cohort (n = 46,704) and found a non-linear relationship between BMI, mental health, and health-adverse behaviors. Obese subjects had significantly greater odds of having mental health illnesses. The data was retrieved from the South Australian Monitoring and Surveillance System and computer assisted telephone interviews were used to collect information on health behavior and suicidal ideation [35].

Impact of Depression on Voice in FM Patients

There are no studies on the impact of depression on voice in FM patients. Although the current literature indicates that FM increases the risk for voice disorders, no study investigated the correlation between dysphonia in FM patients and mental illnesses such as anxiety and depression [17, 36–38]. There are however many reports on the strong link between anxiety, depression and voice. This is in alignment with the general consensus that voice is a reflection of our mental wellbeing and an acoustic cue to our emotions. Anxiety and depression carry a large burden on various systems in the body including the phonatory system. Patients with anxiety and or depression are known to exhibit changes in prosody of speech, intonation and many acoustic features. *Zhao et al.* examined the vocal characteristics of 71 patients with depression and noted a significant difference in all acoustic parameters in comparison to controls. The authors suggested using acoustic features as biomarkers for screening and identification of depression in suspected subjects [39]. The utility of vocal biomarkers in assessing mental health was further evaluated by *Larsen et al.* who devised a "Mental Fitness Vocal Biomarker" (MFVB) which included several vocal features. The results showed that MFVB is a reliable tool to diagnose and stratify the severity of patients' mental condition [40]. Looking at the other side of the coin, patients with voice disorders are also at a higher risk of having mental illnesses. Studies have shown a significantly higher prevalence of anxiety and depression in patients with functional, neurologic and structural voice disorders, with a higher prevalence being noted in those with neurologic disorders [41]. *Maksimovic et al.* investigated the prevalence of anxiety and depression in 205 patients with benign lesions of the vocal folds and noted the presence of mild-to-severe depression and mild-to-moderate anxiety in 38.6% and 97.1% of the cases, respectively [42]. *Cobanoglu et al.* examined the psychological symptoms of patients with vocal fold nodules and found higher Beck Anxiety inventory and Brief Symptom inventory scores in comparison to controls [43]. In a systematic review looking at the psychological characteristics of patients with voice disorders, *Aldridge-Waddon* et al. noted a higher prevalence of self-reported signs of depression, trait and state anxiety in comparison to controls. The authors stressed the need to account for the psychological needs of patients with voice disorders [44]. In another scoping review on the intersection between voice disorders and mental health, *Ravi et al.* reported anxiety and mood disorders in 78.8% and 71.2% of the cases, respectively. The study groups of 156 articles included patients with globus, patients with dysphonia and patients with dysphonia and globus [45].

There are no studies on the impact of mental illnesses on voice in FM patients. However, numerous reports indicate that anxiety and depression impact voice and affected patients have distinctive voice characteristics. By extrapolation, one can fairly assume that FM patients with history of mental illnesses are at a higher risk of having voice disorders in comparison to FM patients with no mental illnesses. Future studies on the correlation between anxiety, depression and dysphonia in patients with FM are needed.

References

1. Vercoulen JH, Swanink CM, Fennis JF, et al. Dimensional assessment of chronic fatigue syndrome. J Psychosom Res. 1994;38:383–92.
2. King C, Jason LA. Improving the diagnostic criteria and procedures for chronic fatigue syndrome. Biol Psychol. 2005;68:87–8106.
3. Bierl C, Nisenbaum R, Hoaglin DC, Randall B, Jones AB, Unger ER, Reeves WC. Regional distribution of fatiguing illnesses in the United States: a pilot study. Popul Health Metrics. 2004;2:1–7.
4. Reeves WC, Jones JF, Maloney E, Heim C, Hoaglin DC, Boneva RS, Morrissey M, Devlin R. Prevalence of chronic fatigue syndrome in metropolitan, urban, and rural Georgia. Popul Health Metrics. 2007;5:5.
5. Mawle AC, Nisenbaum R, Dobbins JG, et al. Seroepidemiology of chronic fatigue syndrome: a case-control study. Clin Infect Dis. 1995;21(6):1386–9.
6. Vercoulen JH, Swanink CM, Fennis JF, Galama JM, van der Meer JW, Bleijenberg G. Dimensional assessment of chronic fatigue syndrome. J Psychosom Res. 1994;38(5):383–92.
7. Reeves WC, Wagner D, Nisenbaum R, Jones JF, Gurbaxani B, Solomon L, Papanicolaou DA, Unger ER, Vernon SD, Heim C. Chronic fatigue syndrome—a clinically empirical approach to its definition and study. BMC Med. 2005;3:1–9.

8. Sharpe MC, Archard LC, Banatvala JE, et al. A report—chronic fatigue syndrome: guidelines for research. J R Soc Med. 1991;84:118–21.
9. Van Houdenhove B, Kempke S, Luyten P. Psychiatric aspects of chronic fatigue syndrome and fibromyalgia. Curr Psychiatry Rep. 2010;12(3):208–14.
10. Bennett R. Fibromyalgia, chronic fatigue syndrome, and myofascial pain. Curr Opin Rheumatol. 1998;10(2):95–103.
11. Bourke JH, Wodehouse T, Clark LV, Constantinou E, Kidd BL, Langford R, Mehta V, White PD. Central sensitisation in chronic fatigue syndrome and fibromyalgia: a case control study. J Psychosom Res. 2021;150:110624.
12. Whistler T, Jones JF, Unger ER, Vernon SD. Exercise responsive genes measured in peripheral blood of women with chronic fatigue syndrome and matched control subjects. BMC Physiol. 2005;5(1):5.
13. Zhang L, Gough J, Christmas D, et al. Microbial infections in eight genomic subtypes of chronic fatigue syndrome/myalgic encephalomyelitis. J Clin Pathol. 2010;63(2):156–64.
14. Chalder T, Godfrey E, Ridsdale L, King M, Wessely S. Predictors of outcome in a fatigued population in primary care following a randomized controlled trial. Psychol Med. 2003;33(2):283–7.
15. Cevik R, Gur A, Acar S, Nas K, Sarac AJ. Hypothalamic-pituitary-gonadal axis hormones and cortisol in both menstrual phases of women with chronic fatigue syndrome and effect of depressive mood on these hormones. BMC Musculoskelet Disord. 2004;5:1–6.
16. Cleare AJ, Miell J, Heap E, et al. Hypothalamo-pituitaryadrenal axis dysfunction in chronic fatigue syndrome, and the effects of low-dose hydrocortisone therapy. J Clin Endocrinol Metab. 2001;86(8):3545–54.
17. Piersiala K, Akst LM, Hillel AT, Best SR. Chronic pain syndromes and their laryngeal manifestations. JAMA Otolaryngol Head Neck Surg. 2020;146(6):543–9.
18. Thoret E, Andrillon T, Gauriau C, Léger D, Pressnitzer D. Sleep deprivation detected by voice analysis. PLoS Comput Biol. 2024;20(2):e1011849.
19. Icht M, Zukerman G, Hershkovich S, Laor T, Heled Y, Fink N, Fostick L. The “morning voice”: the effect of 24 hours of sleep deprivation on vocal parameters of young adults. J Voice. 2020;34(3):489.e1–9.
20. Rocha BR, Behlau M. The influence of sleep disorders on voice quality. J Voice. 2018;32(6):771.e1–771.e13.
21. Helou LB, Wang W, Ashmore RC, Rosen CA, Abbott KV. Intrinsic laryngeal muscle activity in response to autonomic nervous system activation. Laryngoscope. 2013;123(11):2756–65.
22. MacPherson MK, Abur D, Stepp CE. Acoustic measures of voice and physiologic measures of autonomic arousal during speech as a function of cognitive load. J Voice. 2017;31(4):504.e1–9.
23. Park CK, Lee S, Park HJ, Baik YS, Park YB, Park YJ. Autonomic function, voice, and mood states. Clin Auton Res. 2011;21(2):103–10.
24. Ranasinghe KG, Gill JS, Kothare H, Beagle AJ, Mizuiri D, Honma SM, Gorno-Tempini ML, Miller BL, Vossel KA, Nagarajan SS, Houde JF. Abnormal vocal behavior predicts executive and memory deficits in Alzheimer’s disease. Neurobiol Aging. 2017;52:71–80.
25. Galvez-Sánchez CM, Duschek S, Reyes Del Paso GA. Psychological impact of fibromyalgia: current perspectives. Psychol Res Behav Manag. 2019;12:117–27.
26. Campos RP, Vázquez I, Vilhena E. Psychological factors and health-related quality of life in fibromyalgia patients. Health Psychol Rep. 2024;12(4):352–67.
27. Thieme K, Turk DC, Flor H. Comorbid depression and anxiety in fibromyalgia syndrome: relationship to somatic and psychosocial variables. Psychosom Med. 2004;66(6):837–44.
28. Fietta P, Fietta P, Manganelli P. Fibromyalgia and psychiatric disorders. Acta Biomed. 2007;78(2):88–95.
29. Alzabibi MA, Shibani M, Alsuliman T, Ismail H, Alasaad S, Torbey A, Altorkmani A, Sawaf B, Ayoub R, Khalayli N, Kudsi M. Fibromyalgia: epidemiology and risk factors, a population-based case-control study in Damascus, Syria. BMC Rheumatol. 2022;6(1):62.

30. Sadr S, Mobini M, Tabarestani M, Islami Parkoohi P, Elyasi F. The frequency of psychiatric disorder co-morbidities in patients with fibromyalgia: a cross-sectional study in Iran. Nurs Open. 2023;10(7):4797–805.
31. Gardoki-Souto I, Redolar-Ripoll D, Fontana M, et al. Prevalence and characterization of psychological trauma in patients with fibromyalgia: a cross-sectional study. Pain Res Manag. 2022;2022:2114451.
32. Arnaud AM, Brister TS, Duckworth K, et al. Impact of treating depression on associated comorbidities: a systematic literature review. Prim Care Companion CNS Disord. 2023;25(1):44925.
33. Aparicio VA, Ortega FB, Carbonell-Baeza A, Camiletti D, Ruiz JR, Delgado-Fernández M. Relationship of weight status with mental and physical health in female fibromyalgia patients. Obes Facts. 2011;4(6):443–8.
34. Marcus DA. Obesity and the impact of chronic pain. Clin J Pain. 2004;20(3):186–91.
35. Kelly SJ, Daniel M, Dal Grande E, Taylor A. Mental ill-health across the continuum of body mass index. BMC Public Health. 2011;11:1.
36. Hamdan AL, Hosri J, Yammine Y, Ghzayel L, Hadi J, Moussawi MA, Romanos M, Nader N, Uthman I. Voice disorders in patients with fibromyalgia: case series and review of the literature. J Voice. 2024; https://doi.org/10.1016/j.jvoice.2024.06.027.
37. Gurbuzler L, Inanir A, Yelken K, Koc S, Eyibilen A, Uysal IO. Voice disorder in patients with fibromyalgia. Auris Nasus Larynx. 2013;40(6):554–7.
38. Basar G, Kaleoglu Aslan O, Surmeli M. Relationship between dysphonia and anxiety in fibromyalgia syndrome. Eur Arch Otorrinolaringol. 2023;280(1):285–8.
39. Zhao Q, Fan HZ, Li YL, Liu L, Wu YX, Zhao YL, Tian ZX, Wang ZR, Tan YL, Tan SP. Vocal acoustic features as potential biomarkers for identifying/diagnosing depression: a cross-sectional study. Front Psych. 2022;13:815678.
40. Larsen E, Murton O, Song X, Joachim D, Watts D, Kapczinski F, Venesky L, Hurowitz G. Validating the efficacy and value proposition of mental fitness vocal biomarkers in a psychiatric population: prospective cohort study. Front Psych. 2024;15:1342835.
41. White LJ, Hapner ER, Klein AM, Delgaudio JM, Hanfelt JJ, Jinnah HA, Johns MM III. Coprevalence of anxiety and depression with spasmodic dysphonia: a case-control study. J Voice. 2012;26(5):667–e1.
42. Maksimovic JM, Vukasinovic MM, Vlajinac HD, Jotic AD, Milovanovic MS, Ivanov SY, Maksimovic MZ, Milovanovic JP. Anxiety and depression in patients with vocal fold nodules, edema and polyps. Eur Arch Otorrinolaringol. 2020;277(9):2493–500.
43. Çobanoglu HB, Ogut MF, Sirin S, Arslan FC. The evaluation of beck anxiety scale, voice handicap index, and brief symptom inventory on treatment of patients with vocal fold nodules. J Voice. 2023;37(3):470.e1–6.
44. Aldridge-Waddon L, Hiles C, Spence V, Hotton M. Clinical psychology and voice disorders: a meta-analytic review of studies assessing psychological characteristics across individuals with and without voice disorders. J Voice. 2023; https://doi.org/10.1016/j.jvoice.2023.09.012.
45. Ravi S, Lopez V, Carter KV, Sharpe SA, George D, Ebersole B, Machiorlatti M, Jamal N. Intersection of mental health and dysphonia: a scoping review. J Voice. 2023; https://doi.org/10.1016/j.jvoice.2023.04.007.

Obesity in Patients with Fibromyalgia and Its Impact on Voice

14

Abdul-latif Hamdan, Robert Thayer Sataloff, and Mary J. Hawkshaw

Prevalence of Obesity in Fibromyalgia

Fibromyalgia (FM) is a chronic neuromuscular syndrome associated with a number of co-morbidities among which is obesity. Numerous studies indicate a strong epidemiologic link between FM and obesity. In a retrospective analysis which included 411 participants, Rivera et al. noted the prevalence of obesity in 18.2% of their study group. Other co-morbidities included hypothyroidism and osteoarthritis [1]. Bennett et al. conducted an internet survey on 2569 patients with FM and noted obesity in 43% and overweight in more than two-thirds of the cases. The authors stressed on the role of behavioral modification in addressing co-morbidities of FM among which is obesity [2]. Okifuji et al. reported a positive correlation between BMI and neuroendocrine biomarkers, namely epinephrine and IL-6 ($r = 0.54$ and $r = 0.52$, respectively) in a cohort of FM patients 50% of whom were obese [3]. Aparicio et al. analyzed the body composition of 104 women with FM and found a mean body mass index (BMI) of 28.6 + 5.1 kg/m^2, and a mean body fat mass of 38.6 + 7.6% [4]. In another study of 177 females diagnosed with FM, Aparacio et al. noted the prevalence of overweight/obesity in 70% of the cases. The authors stressed the high prevalence of obesity in patients with FM [5].

What is more interesting is the significant correlation between weight status and the severity of symptoms in affected patients. Neumann et al. conducted a cross-sectional study on patients with FM and reported a negative correlation between BMI, tenderness threshold and quality of life ($r = -0.238$ and $r = -0.205$, respectively). More than two thirds of their study group (73%) were either obese or overweight [6]. Yunus et al. investigated the relationship between BMI and Fibromyalgia in 211 patients presenting to a rheumatology clinic and found a trend for mild significance in the correlation between obesity and number of

A.-l. Hamdan et al., *Voice Disorders in Fibromyalgia*,
https://doi.org/10.1007/978-3-031-97751-0_14

tender points and fatigue. Moreover, there was a significant correlation between BMI and the Health Assessment Questionnaire score [7]. Aparicio et al. examined the relationship between weight status, bodily pain and physical functioning in a cohort of 175 patients with Fibromyalgia and reported worse SF36 scores across the different weight categories [8]. Kim et al. assessed the correlation between BMI and symptom severity in 888 patients with FM using the Fibromyalgia Impact Questionnaire and noted significant worsening of symptoms and pain with an increase in BMI [9]. Atzeni et al. analyzed the relationship between BMI and symptom severity in 2339 patients with FM who were stratified according to their BMI and noted that the overweight/obese group had more impairment in symptomatology and function than the underweight group. The authors used the Fibromyalgia Impact Questionnaire in addition to the Polysymptomatic Distress Scale and the modified Fibromyalgia Assessment Status questionnaire. It is worth noting that the obese/overweight subgroup constituted 51.8% of the total group [10].

All the above confirms that obesity is a comorbidity in patients with FM. There is also a positive correlation between BMI, severity of pain and number of tenderness points. Obese and overweight FM patients are more likely to experience impairment in bodily activity and daily function.

Why the Overlap Between Obesity and Fibromyalgia

The epidemiologic link between obesity and Fibromyalgia is a subject of thorough debate in the literature. The most accepted hypotheses are diffuse musculoskeletal pain and the high rate of inactivity and or disability in obese patients.

The Musculoskeletal Pain in Obesity and Fibromyalgia

Musculoskeletal pain, be it diffuse or localized, is a common symptom in obese subjects. In a study which included 6328 obese patients, Peltonen et al. reported an increased odds of self-reported work-restricting pain in the back, hip, neck, knee and ankle in comparison to controls [11]. Bingefors et al. conducted a cross sectional study looking at the prevalence of musculoskeletal pain in the general population and noted an association between pain and obesity, in addition to other psychological and other socio-economic factors. The most common type of pain were back pain and shoulder pain noted in 22.7% and 21.0% of their study population [12]. Holmberg et al. investigated the risk of knee osteoarthritis in relation to BMI and reported a fourfold increase in men with a BMI between 23 and 25 kg/m^2 in comparison to those with a BMI less than 23 kg/m^2. In women, the odd ratio was 1.6 with a confidence interval of 96% [13]. Shiri et al. reported a high prevalence of back pain in women with a high BMI and high waist-to-hip ratio among other anthropometric measures. The odds of having low back pain in women increased 1.8 times in those with a waist circumference greater than or equal to 88 cm in comparison to those with a waist circumference less than 88 cm [14]. The same authors also conducted a meta-analysis on the association between obesity and low back pain which included cross-sectional and cohort studies. The cross-sectional studies showed that the odds of having low back pain over the past 1 year and the odds of seeking care for that pain in obese subjects were 1.33 and 1.56, respectively. Cohort studies also showed an association between obesity and low back pain with a higher incidence of having low back pain for more than 1 day over the last 12 months in obese subjects compared to non-obese subjects [15].

What further substantiates the strong correlation between obesity and musculoskeletal pain is the decrease in pain following weight reduction. Hooper et al. investigated musculoskeletal pain in 48 obese patients (mean BMI of 51 + 8 kg/m^2) undergoing bariatric surgery and reported a significant decrease in the severity of pain after weight loss (mean 41 + 15 kg). Before surgery, all patients had lower extremities musculoskeletal pain and 79% had upper extremities musculoskeletal pain [16]. Peltonen et al. reported a decrease in the severity of pain in the knee and ankle following a decrease in weight after bariatric surgery in a large group of obese patients who were followed-up for 2-years after surgical intervention [11]. Felson et al. investigated the effect of weight loss on the prevalence of symptomatic osteoarthritis and noted that a decrease of 5.1 kg over the course of 10 years resulted in a 50% decrease in the odds of having osteoarthritis (p value 0.02) [17]. In a study group of 80 obese patients (BMI =35.9 kg/m^2) with knee osteoarthritis, Christensen et al. reported that a 10% decrease in weight led to a 28% improvement in knee function. For each 1% reduction n percent of body fat, there was a 9.4% improvement in the Western Ontario and McMaster Universities (WOMAC) osteoarthritis index [18].

Why do obese subjects suffer from diffuse pain? Numerous studies in the literature indicate that obesity is associated with a persistent low-grade inflammation. This state of chronic inflammation is associated with systemic complaints among which is pain. This is not surprising given that adipose tissue is known to secrete a large range of pro-inflammatory cytokines that are sensitizers of many inflammatory markers connected to pain sensation, such as C-reactive protein (CRP) [19]. Elevation in the levels of inflammatory markers is suggestive of a chronic inflammatory state that can partially be responsible for the diffuse and/or localized pain in obese subjects. Su et al. conducted a systematic review on inflammatory markers in relation to obesity and noted higher levels of CRP and interleukin-6 (IL-6) in metabolically unhealthy obese in comparison to metabolically healthy obese. There was no statistically significant difference in tumor necrosis factor-alpha (TNF-alpha) between metabolically healthy obese and metabolically unhealthy obese [20]. Hainsworth et al. examined the levels of circulating inflammatory biomarkers in a multiple-cohort observational study and noted the highest levels of IL-6 and CRP in the subgroup of obese patients with chronic pain in comparison to obese patients with no pain, and non-obese patients. The high level of these markers was also associated with functional disability [21]. Siefkaste al investigated the association between inflammatory markers and foot pain in 909 patients with known foot disorders and noted an association between CRP, foot pain and forefoot pain even after adjusting for confounding factors. A similar association was reported in regard to IL-6 [22].

The high prevalence of diffuse musculoskeletal pain in obese patients may mask the diagnosis of FM given that widespread body ache is a cardinal symptom of this syndrome. On the other hand, diffuse pain in FM patients with high BMI should raise suspicion whether obesity is a main precipitating factor. Physicians should be alert that obesity and FM are not mutually exclusive and that obese patients suffering from diffuse body pain need to be investigated about FM.

Inactivity and Deconditioning in Obesity and Fibromyalgia

The second link between obesity and Fibromyalgia is the sedentary behavior commonly observed in obese and FM patients. Both obesity and FM are associated with a decrease in physical activity and deconditioning, which create a vicious cycle that feeds into the morbidity of each of these conditions. Marcus et al. conducted a survey on disability and pain severity in 372 patients with a history of chronic pain and noted a positive correlation between BMI and reduced activity. An increase in body weight resulted in an increase in disability. The authors concluded that obesity is a potential marker of disability and a comorbid condition in subjects with chronic pain [23]. Inactivity and decrease in functional capacity in obese patients may be a predisposing factor for FM. Mork et al. investigated the risk of FM in relation to physical exercise in a large female population (n = 15,990) and noted a dose-response association (r = 0.13), although weak, between the risk of FM and degree of exercise. Those who exercised heavily were less likely to develop FM [24].

Looking at the other side of the coin, FM is also a predisposing factor for inactivity and decrease in exercise tolerance. In a study on the impact of associated comorbidities on FM treatment, Rivera et al. reported an association between obesity and the risk of functional impairment. Obese participants had a higher risk of impairment in comparison to non-obese [1]. In a study on 38 patients diagnosed with FM, Okifuji et al. noted a negative correlation between BMI and distance walked (r = −0.41) [3]. In a study which included 100 patients, Neumann et al. reported a positive correlation between BMI and physical deconditioning (r = 0.202). Moreover, an increase in weight led to dysfunction and worsening in quality of life [6]. Aparicio et al. compared the level of fatigue in relation to weight status in a cohort of female patients with FM and found a positive correlation between BMI, fatigue and tiredness. In addition, obese and overweight subjects had significantly more stiffness [5]. In a systematic review on the level of physical activity in patients with FM, Vancampfort et al. reported that patients with FM had less vigorous physical activity per week in comparison to controls (5663.7 vs. 6000 steps per day, respectively). Close to one third (37.7%) achieved the recommended public physical activity needed for a good health [25]. In another systematic review by the same group, the authors noted that patients with FM spent more sedentary time (36.14 min) compared to the general population. The authors highlighted the association between decrease in physical activity and severity of disease in terms of pain and fatigue [26]. Gavilan-Carrera et al. conducted a longitudinal study on the predictive value of physical activity and sedentary time on pain and quality of life in 427 patients diagnosed with FM and noted that increasing moderate-to-vigorous activity at baseline and reducing sedentary time resulted in a decrease in bodily pain over the course of 5-years. Moreover, an increase in light physical activity was also associated with improvement in health-related quality of life [27].

In summary, it is not clear if the widespread musculoskeletal pain in FM results in a decrease in physical activity thus leading to weight gain, or whether obesity leads to reduced activity which in turn increases pain sensitivity and body aches. The cross-cutting between weight gain secondary to deconditioning in FM patients and pain secondary to reduced activity in obese patients remains a mystery.

Impact of Obesity on Voice in Patients with Fibromyalgia

There are no studies in the literature on the impact of obesity on voice in patients with FM but there are many reports on the voice characteristics of obese subjects.

Prevalence of Voice Disorders in Obese Patients

There is ubiquity of reports in the literature on voice characteristics of obese patients. In 2011, da Cunha et al. reported that subjects with a BMI above 35 kg/m^2 had more hoarseness and strangulation at the end of sound emission than subjects with a BMI less than 30 kg/m^2. Moreover, they had higher perturbation parameters, namely jitter and shimmer, and a shorter MPT in comparison to a control group of patients with BMI below 30 kg/m^2 [28]. In 2011, Solomon et al. conducted a longitudinal study on eight obese patients who underwent bariatric surgery and noted a significant decrease in phonatory threshold pressure (PTP) at comfortable pitch and at 30% and 80% of the frequency range following treatment. On the other hand, there was no significant difference in any of the pre-operative subjective or objective voice measures during sustained vowel between obese patients and controls [29]. In 2013, Celebi et al. investigated the vocal characteristics of 20 obese subjects in comparison to a control group of 20 normal weight volunteers and noted a significant difference in auditory perceptual evaluation between the two groups. Although obese subjects had lower maximum phonation time (19.6 + 4.9 s vs. 26.4 + 4.1 s), there was no significant difference in self-perceived hoarseness or in any of the acoustic parameters between the two groups [30]. In 2014, Acurio et al. investigated the impact of vocal loading on acoustic parameters in normal weight, overweight and obese school teachers. The results showed a significant elevation in the fundamental frequency (Fo) in the obese group and a significant increase in IL-6 in the overweight group [31]. In 2015, in a longitudinal study on a cohort of 21 morbidly obese women, Rocha de Souza reported the presence of vocal complaints in 2/3 of the cases, most common of which were vocal fatigue, vocal failure and increase in vocal effort. All these symptoms improved after bariatric surgery [32]. In 2018, Rocha de Souza conducted acoustic analysis on subjects with different weight status and noted significant differences in F0 and MPT across the subgroups. The authors concluded that an increase in BMI had an impact on vocal pitch and duration of sustained phonation [33]. In 2021, Bosso et al. compared the vocal characteristics of 27 obese subjects and 27 ideal weight controls and noted more hoarseness, roughness, breathiness and voice instability in the obese group. These vocal characteristics were associated with laryngeal edema and hyperemia on endoscopic examination. The authors ascribed the laryngeal findings to gastroesophageal reflux disease [34]. In 2024, Munjal et al. conducted a perceptual, acoustic and aerodynamic evaluation of 40 obese participants and found a significantly higher normalized noise energy and F0 in the study group in comparison to 40 non-obese subjects. Moreover, the obese group had a shorter MPT and reduced expiratory reserve volume compared to controls [35].

The Pathophysiology of Voice Changes in Obese Patients

The pathophysiology of voice disorders of obese subjects is very complex. Several mechanisms have been suggested: One is the change in vocal tract (VT) shape and dimension. The vocal tract morphology is a major determinant of voice timber. A change in vocal tract morphology impacts the position and dispersion of these formants leading to a change in voice quality [36–38]. Obese patients are known to have distinctive anatomic variations in their vocal tract shape and length. Using radiologic imaging, Horner et al. reported excess fat deposition at different sites of the vocal tract in obese patients, mostly at the palatopharyngeal area and base of tongue [39]. Obese patients with and without obstructive sleep apnea have also been shown to have larger neck tissue volume in comparison to non-obese subjects. The difference is mostly ascribed to fat deposition in the retroglossal and retropalatal areas [40]. Similarly, individuals with high BMI have been shown to have enlargement of the base of tongue and thickening of the nasopharyngeal tissues leading to narrowing of the airway. The soft tissue changes noted in obese patients are often associated with variations in the laryngeal skeletal architecture such as antero-inferior displacement of the hyoid bone [41]. There are also studies supporting a link between VT length and obesity. Roers et al. reported a significant correlation between the length of the vocal tract and body weight in a cohort of 34 subjects [30]. Similarly, Schen et al. reported a positive correlation between body weight and nasopharyngeal tract length ($r = 0.81$) [42].

Obesity can also affect voice the power source of phonation, the respiratory system. It is well established that dyspnea and shortness of breath are common complaints in obese subjects even in the absence of pulmonary diseases [43]. Obesity has been shown to be a predictor of breathlessness which also correlates with the rate of perceived exertion [44, 45]. In a study which included 23 obese patients with a BMI greater than 28 kg/m^2, the prevalence of dyspnea was noted in 65% of the study group [46]. The symptoms of dyspnea and breathlessness are often associated with abnormal pulmonary function testing. Many studies documented limitations in expiratory flow, decrease in FEV1, vital capacity and functional residual capacity in obese subjects in comparison to normal weight subjects [47–54]. These respiratory changes are not associated only with the level of BMI but also with type of fat distribution. Android type of obesity has worse effect on breathing than the genoid type. Chen et al. reported that with a 1 cm increase in waist circumference, there is a 13 ml decrease in forced vital capacity [55]. The changes in respiration in obese subjects have been attributed to several factors: One is mechanical impairment with restriction in the downward movement of the diaphragm as a result of the excess fat deposition in the abdomen. This ineffective diaphragmatic contraction correlates with dyspnea score and with disturbances in phonation [56]. Other causes of respiratory changes in obese subjects include a decrease in chest wall compliance which often leads to increase in mechanical work of breathing [57]. alteration in lung ventilation and perfusion [58, 59], alteration in respiratory neural drive and breathing pattern [60]. All of these factors can affect voice given the paramount role of breathing in phonation. In a study on the impact of respiratory rate on voice, Sandage et al. reported that breathing for 8 min at a respiratory rate of 20 per minute can lead to an increase in the phonatory threshold pressure which in turn correlates with phonatory effort [61].

Another factor by which obesity can impact voice is the change in sex hormones concentration. Obesity affects sex hormones in both genders, before and after puberty. There are numerous reports in the literature indicating that an increase in adipose tissue leads to an increase in estradiol and estrone [62–66]. The increase in estrogen in turns affects the concentration and distribution of fat via both peripheral and central pathways. Suggested mechanisms include alteration in adipose tissue blood supply, increase in metabolic rate, activation in estrogen receptors and modulation in the activity of the limbic-pituitary adrenal axis [67–72]. Obesity has also been associated with low testosterone level. The low levels are partially ascribed to the conversion of testosterone in the adipose tissue to estrogen via cytochrome P450 [73]. Moreover, fat distribution in addition to its concentration also affects the level of testosterone. Given that obesity tempers sex hormone concentration and that the larynx is a hormonal target with the presence of sex hormone receptors in various laryngeal structures [74–76], it is intuitive that obesity affects voice.

References

1. Rivera FA, Munipalli B, Allman ME, et al. A retrospective analysis of the prevalence and impact of associated comorbidities on fibromyalgia outcomes in a tertiary care center. Front Med (Lausanne). 2024;10:1301944.
2. Bennett RM, Jones J, Turk DC, et al. An internet survey of 2,596 people with fibromyalgia. BMC Musculoskelet Disord. 2007;8:1–1.
3. Okifuji A, Bradshaw DH, Olson C. Evaluating obesity in fibromyalgia: neuroendocrine biomarkers, symptoms, and functions. Clin Rheumatol. 2009;28(4):475–8.
4. Aparicio VA, Ortega FB, Heredia JM, et al. Análisis de la composición corporal en mujeres con fibromialgia [Analysis of the body composition of Spanish women with fibromyalgia]. Reumatol Clin. 2011;7(1):7–12.
5. Aparicio VA, Segura-Jiménez V, Alvarez-Gallardo IC, et al. Are there differences in quality of life, symptomatology and functional capacity among different obesity classes in women with fibromyalgia? The al-Ándalus project. Rheumatol Int. 2014;34(6):811–21.
6. Neumann L, Lerner E, Glazer Y, et al. A cross-sectional study of the relationship between body mass index and clinical characteristics, tenderness measures, quality of life, and physical functioning in fibromyalgia patients. Clin Rheumatol. 2008;27(12):1543–7.
7. Yunus MB, Arslan S, Aldag JC. Relationship between body mass index and fibromyalgia features. Scand J Rheumatol. 2002;31(1):27–31.
8. Aparicio VA, Ortega FB, Carbonell-Baeza A, Camiletti D, Ruiz JR, Delgado-Fernández M. Relationship of weight status with mental and physical health in female fibromyalgia patients. Obes Facts. 2011;4(6):443–8.
9. Kim CH, Luedtke CA, Vincent A, Thompson JM, Oh TH. Association of body mass index with symptom severity and quality of life in patients with fibromyalgia. Arthritis Care Res (Hoboken). 2012;64(2):222–8.
10. Atzeni F, Alciati A, Salaffi F, et al. The association between body mass index and fibromyalgia severity: data from a cross-sectional survey of 2339 patients. Rheumatol Adv Pract. 2021;5(1):rkab015.
11. Peltonen M, Lindroos AK, Torgerson JS. Musculoskeletal pain in the obese: a comparison with a general population and long-term changes after conventional and surgical obesity treatment. Pain. 2003;104(3):549–57.
12. Bingefors K, Isacson D. Epidemiology, co-morbidity, and impact on health-related quality of life of self-reported headache and musculoskeletal pain—a gender perspective. Eur J Pain. 2004;8(5):435–50.
13. Holmberg S, Thelin A, Thelin N. Knee osteoarthritis and body mass index: a population-based case-control study. Scand J Rheumatol. 2005;34(1):59–64.
14. Shiri R, Solovieva S, Husgafvel-Pursiainen K, et al. The association between obesity and the prevalence of low back pain in young adults: the cardiovascular risk in young Finns study. Am J Epidemiol. 2008;167(9):1110–9.
15. Shiri R, Karppinen J, Leino-Arjas P, et al. The association between obesity and low back pain: a meta-analysis. Am J Epidemiol. 2010;171(2):135–54.
16. Hooper MM, Stellato TA, Hallowell PT, et al. Musculoskeletal findings in obese subjects before and after weight loss following bariatric surgery. Int J Obes. 2007;31(1):114–20.
17. Felson DT, Zhang Y, Anthony JM, et al. Weight loss reduces the risk for symptomatic knee osteoarthritis in women. The Framingham study. Ann Intern Med. 1992;116(7):535–9.
18. Christensen R, Astrup A, Bliddal H. Weight loss: the treatment of choice for knee osteoarthritis? A randomized trial. Osteoarthritis Cartilage. 2005;13(1):20–7.
19. da Cruz Fernandes IM, Pinto RZ, Ferreira P, Lira FS. Low back pain, obesity, and inflammatory markers: exercise as potential treatment. J Exerc Rehabil. 2018;14(2):168–74.
20. Su Z, Efremov L, Mikolajczyk R. Differences in the levels of inflammatory markers between metabolically healthy obese and other obesity phenotypes in adults: a systematic review and meta-analysis. Nutr Metab Cardiovasc Dis. 2024;34(2):251–69.

21. Hainsworth KR, Simpson PM, Raff H, et al. Circulating inflammatory biomarkers in adolescents: evidence of interactions between chronic pain and obesity. Pain Rep. 2021;6(1):e916.
22. Siefkas AC, Dufour AB, Golightly YM, et al. Foot pain and inflammatory markers: a cross sectional study in older adults. J Foot Ankle Res. 2022;15(1):57.
23. Marcus DA. Obesity and the impact of chronic pain. Clin J Pain. 2004;20(3):186–91.
24. Mork PJ, Vasseljen O, Nilsen TI. Association between physical exercise, body mass index, and risk of fibromyalgia: longitudinal data from the Norwegian Nord-Trøndelag Health Study. Arthritis Care Res (Hoboken). 2010;62(5):611–7.
25. Vancampfort D, Van Damme T, McGrath RL, et al. Physical activity levels among people with fibromyalgia: a systematic review and meta-analysis. Musculoskeletal Care. 2023;21(3):623–32.
26. Vancampfort D, Van Damme T, Albanio Machado V, et al. Levels of sedentary behaviour in people with fibromyalgia: a systematic review and meta-analysis. Disabil Rehabil. 2024;46(10):1921–7.
27. Gavilán-Carrera B, Delgado-Fernández M, Álvarez-Gallardo IC, et al. Longitudinal association of sedentary time and physical activity with pain and quality of life in fibromyalgia. Scand J Med Sci Sports. 2023;33(3):292–306.
28. da Cunha MG, Passerotti GH, Weber R, et al. Voice feature characteristic in morbid obese population. Obes Surg. 2011;21(3):340–4.
29. Solomon NP, Helou LB, Dietrich-Burns K, et al. Do obesity and weight loss affect vocal function? Semin Speech Lang. 2011;32(1):31–42.
30. Celebi S, Yelken K, Develioglu ON, et al. Acoustic, perceptual and aerodynamic voice evaluation in an obese population. J Laryngol Otol. 2013;127(10):987–90.
31. Acurio J, Celis C, Perez J, et al. Acoustic parameters and salivary IL-6 levels in overweight and obese teachers. J Voice. 2014;28(5):574–81.
32. de Souza LB, Pernambuco Lde A, dos Santos MM, et al. Vocal complaint, auditory-perceptual assessment of voice and vocal self-assessment in women with morbid obesity. Arq Bras Cir Dig. 2015;28((Suppl 1)):23–5.
33. de Souza LBR, Dos Santos MM, Pernambuco LA, et al. Effects of weight loss on acoustic parameters after bariatric surgery. Obes Surg. 2018;28(5):1372–6.
34. Bosso JR, Martins RHG, Pessin ABB, et al. Vocal characteristics of patients with morbid obesity. J Voice. 2021;35(2):329.e7–329.e11.
35. Munjal S, Sharma A, Chhabra N, Panda N. Perceptual, aerodynamic and acoustic evaluation of vocal characteristics in subjects with obesity. J Voice. 2024;38(3):660–5.
36. Roers F, Mürbe D, Sundberg J. Voice classification and vocal tract of singers: a study of x-ray images and morphology. JASA. 2009;125(1):503–12.
37. Cleveland TF. Acoustic properties of voice timbre types and their influence on voice classification. JASA. 1977;61(6):1622–9.
38. Dmitriev L, Kiselev A. Relationship between the formant structure of different types of singing voices and the dimensions of supraglottic cavities. Folia Phoniatr. 1979;31(4):238–41.
39. Horner RL, Mohiaddin RH, Lowell DG, et al. Sites and sizes of fat deposits around the pharynx in obese patients with obstructive sleep apnoea and weight matched controls. Eur Respir J. 1989;2(7):613–22.
40. Mortimore IL, Marshall I, Wraith PK, Sellar RJ, Douglas NJ. Neck and total body fat deposition in nonobese and obese patients with sleep apnea compared with that in control subjects. Am J Respir Crit Care Med. 1998;157(1):280–3.
41. Sakakibara H, Tong M, Matsushita K, Hirata M, Konishi Y, Suetsugu S. Cephalometric abnormalities in non-obese and obese patients with obstructive sleep apnoea. Eur Respir J. 1999;13(2):403–10.
42. Shen CM, Soong WJ, Jeng MJ, Lee YS, Cheng CY, Sun J, Hwang B. Nasopharyngeal tract length measurement in infants. Acta Paediatr Taiwan. 2002;43(2):82–5.
43. Bernhardt V, Babb TG. Exertional dyspnoea in obesity. Eur Respir Rev. 2016;25(142):487–95.

44. Bowden JA, To THM, Abernethy AP, Currow DC. Predictors of chronic breathlessness: a large population study. BMC Public Health. 2011;11(1):33.
45. Bernhardt V, Wood HE, Moran RB, Babb TG. Dyspnea on exertion in obese men. Respir Physiol Neurobiol. 2013;185(2):241–8.
46. Sahebjami H. Dyspnea in obese healthy men. Chest. 1988;114(5):1373–7.
47. Dixon AE, Peters U. The effect of obesity on lung function. Expert Rev Respir Med. 2018;12(9):755–67.
48. Leone N, Courbon D, Thomas F, et al. Lung function impairment and metabolic syndrome: the critical role of abdominal obesity. Am J Respir Crit Care Med. 2009;179(6):509–16.
49. Littleton SW. Impact of obesity on respiratory function. Respirology. 2012;17(1):43–9.
50. Jones RL, Nzekwu MMU. The effects of body mass index on lung volumes. Chest. 2006;130(3):827–33.
51. Pelosi P, Croci M, Ravagnan I, et al. The effects of body mass on lung volumes, respiratory mechanics, and gas exchange during general anesthesia. Anesth Analg. 1998;87:654–60.
52. Canoy D, Luben R, Welch A, et al. Abdominal obesity and respiratory function in men and women in the EPIC-Norfolk study, United Kingdom. Am J Epidemiol. 2004;159(12):1140–9.
53. Ray CS, Sue DY, Bray G, Hansen JE, Wasserman K. Effects of obesity on respiratory function. Am Rev Respir Dis. 1983;128(3):501–6.
54. Ofir D, Laveneziana P, Webb KA, O'Donnell DE. Ventilatory and perceptual responses to cycle exercise in obese women. J Appl Physiol. 2007;102(6):2217–26.
55. Chen Y, Rennie D, Cormier YF, Dosman J. Waist circumference is associated with pulmonary function in normal-weight, overweight, and obese subjects. Am J Clin Nutr. 2007;85(1):35–9.
56. Lotti P, Gigliotti F, Tesi F, et al. Respiratory muscles and dyspnea in obese nonsmoking subjects. Lung. 2005;183(5):311–23.
57. Naimark A, Cherniack RM. Compliance of the respiratory system and its components in health and obesity. J Appl Physiol. 1960;15(3):377–82.
58. Milic-Emili J, Torchio R, D'Angelo E. Closing volume: a reappraisal (1967–2007). Eur J Appl Physiol. 2007;99(6):567–83.
59. Hedenstierna G, Santesson J, Norlander O. Airway closure and distribution of inspired gas in the extremely obese, breathing spontaneously and during anaesthesia with intermittent positive pressure ventilation. Acta Anaesthesiol Scand. 1976;20(4):334–42.
60. Chlif M, Keochkerian D, Choquet D, Vaidie A, Ahmaidi S. Effects of obesity on breathing pattern, ventilatory neural drive and mechanics. Respir Physiol Neurobiol. 2009;168(3):198–202.
61. Sandage MJ, Connor NP, Pascoe DD. Voice function differences following resting breathing versus submaximal exercise. J Voice. 2013;27(5):572–8.
62. Glass AR, Swerdloff RS, Bray GA, Dahms WT, Atkinson RL. Low serum testosterone and sex-hormone-binding-globulin in massively obese men. J Clin Endocrinol Metab. 1977;45:1211–9.
63. Amatruda JM, Harman SM, Pourmotabbed G, Lockwood DH. Depressed plasma testosterone and fractional binding of testosterone in obese males. J Clin Endocrinol Metab. 1978;47(2):268–71.
64. Schneider G, Kirschner MA, Berkowitz R, Ertel NH. Increased estrogen production in obese men. J Clin Endocrinol Metab. 1979;48(4):663–8.
65. Kley HK, Solbach HG, McKinnan JC, Kruskemper HL. Testosterone decrease and oestrogen increase in male patients with obesity. Acta Endocrinol. 1979;91:553–63.
66. Bernasconi D, Del Monte P, Meozzi M, Randazzo M, Marugo A, Badaracco B, Marugo M. The impact of obesity on hormonal parameters in hirsute and nonhirsute women. Metabolism. 1996;45(1):72–5.
67. López M, Tena-Sempere M. Estradiol and brown fat. Best Pract Res Clin Endocrinol Metab. 2016;30(4):527–36.

68. Gealekman OL, Guseva N, Hartigan C, Apotheker S, Gorgoglione M, Gurav K, et al. Depot-specific differences and insufficient subcutaneous adipose tissue angiogenesis in human obesity. Circulation. 2011;123:186–94.
69. Nookaew I, Svensson PA, Jacobson P, et al. Adipose tissue resting energy expenditure and expression of genes involved in mitochondrial function are higher in women than in men. J Clin Endocrinol Metab. 2013;98(2):E370–8.
70. Luglio HF. Estrogen and body weight regulation in women: the role of estrogen receptor alpha (ER-α) on adipocyte lipolysis. Acta Med Indones. 2014;46(4):333–8.
71. Michopoulos V. Stress-induced alterations in estradiol sensitivity increase risk for obesity in women. Physiol Behav. 2016;166:56–64.
72. Clegg DJ, Brown LM, Woods SC, Benoit SC. Gonadal hormones determine sensitivity to central leptin and insulin. Diabetes. 2006;55(4):978–87.
73. Kim JH, Cho HT, Kim YJ. The role of estrogen in adipose tissue metabolism: insights into glucose homeostasis regulation. Endocr J. 2014;61(11):1055–67.
74. Newman SR, Butler J, Hammond EH, Gray SD. Preliminary report on hormone receptors in the human vocal fold. J Voice. 2000;14(1):72–81.
75. Tuohimaa PT, Kallio S, Heinijoki J. Androgen receptors in laryngeal carcinoma. Acta Oto-laryngol (Stockholm). 1981;91:149–54.
76. Aufdemorte TB, Sheridan PJ, Holt GR. Autoradiographic evidence of sex steroid receptors in laryngeal tissues of the baboon. Laryngoscope. 1983;93(12):1607–11.

Treatment of Fibromyalgia 15

Abdul-latif Hamdan, Robert Thayer Sataloff,
Mary J. Hawkshaw, and Lana Ghzayel

Non-pharmacologic Treatment of Fibromyalgia

Patient Education

Non-pharmacologic treatment of FM as a syndrome requires patient engagement and collaboration. Patient's motivation and participation are extremely important for optimizing the outcome of any treatment modality. Patient engagement starts with education about the disease, associated comorbidities, and prognosis. Providing insights on the nature of FM and factors contributing to its progress is essential before prior to the initiation of any of treatment strategy. Programs on dietary modification, weight loss, sleep regulation and change in self-perception are recommended often [1].

Another cardinal feature in patient education is the establishment of a baseline. Where does the patient stand in terms of daily exercise and inactivity? What is his or her level of awareness regarding internal and external stressors? These are some of the questions that need to be answered for both the healthcare team and the patient in order to define the starting points before therapy. This process can help ameliorate many of the aggravating factors and even may obviate the need for pharmacologic treatment in many cases [1, 2].

A.-l. Hamdan et al., *Voice Disorders in Fibromyalgia*,
https://doi.org/10.1007/978-3-031-97751-0_15

Cognitive Behavioral Therapy

Cognitive behavioral therapy (CBT) is one of the gold-standard treatment modalities for FM. It is a form of psychotherapy that aims at diminishing negative thought patterns with the purpose of reducing stress and improving a patient's behavior. There is growing evidence supporting the usefulness of CBT and its added value in diminishing perception of pain and in alleviating the negative effects of FM in many patients [1]. In FM, CBT also aims at identifying and restructuring socioemotional burdens and other challenges that compound the severity of symptoms.

The steep rise in the delivery of healthcare services including is CBT has broadened the application of this form of intervention in patients with FM. Based on the recommendations of the European Allies of Association of Rheumatology (EULAR), CBT is advocated as the first line of treatment for FM, and pharmacotherapy is recommended if there is no response to CBT [3]. In a systematic review and meta-analysis on the efficacy and acceptability of CBT in FM, *Benardy et al.* reported that patients treated with CBT had superior results in comparison to those who had no treatment. Cognitive behavioral therapy was found to be successful in relieving pain by 50% or more, in reducing disability and negative mood, and in improving health-related quality of life [4]. *Glombiewski et al.* conducted a meta-analysis on psychological treatments for FM and noted their effectiveness in reducing short-term and long-term pain over a follow-up period of 7.4 months. Moreover, psychological treatments were effective in treating associated comorbidities such as depression and sleep disorders and in reducing catastrophizing pain [5]. In another randomized control study that included 60 FM patients all of whom were treated with amitriptyline and half of whom also received additional CBT, *Falcao D et al.* noted superior results in those treated with combined CBT and pharmacotherapy [6].

Mindfulness-Meditation

Mindfulness-meditation or mindfulness-based intervention (MBI) is gaining ground as an effective treatment alternative for FM. Although the analgesic mechanism behind this mind-body technique needs further understanding, this form of intervention has been shown to improve the clinical course of the disease and patient overall well-being [7]. Mindfulness-meditation is based on cultivating non-reactive sensory awareness that helps attenuate pain via psychological and physiological pathways. By identifying the external and internal stressors, patients learn how to avert them and cope better with their disease. In many instances MBI is coupled with a compassion-based approach to help patient accept their condition better and be less judgmental. Mindefulness-based intervention has evolved over the years from the first generation founded on breathing, meditation and yoga to the second generation that is more holistic, spiritual and focused on non-attachment to self and to the environment [8–10]. In a study that included 74 patients with FM, 8-week training using second generation MBI led to a decrease in pain perception and in psychological distress. The training also resulted in significant improvement in non-attachment and civic engagement. The duration of therapy was predictive of the outcome and extent of improvement [11].

Exercise

Exercise is one of the most recommended non-pharmacologic treatments for FM. Low- intensity and low-impact exercises can help improve the fitness of the patient and reduce various somatic and non-somatic symptoms [12]. Common examples of exercise include stretching, walking, swimming, dancing and simply performing domestic chores that require a low degree of strenuous activity yet keep the patient active. All of these help to reduce rigidity and stiffness, enhancing cardiovascular fitness and improving the overall well being of patients. In a study comparing four self-treatment modalities in 207 FM patients, *Rooks et al.* reported improvement in not only symptoms of FM but also in the functional status and self-efficacy of affected women. The authors also noted that those treated by strength training, aerobic and flexibility exercise had better improvement in their Fibromyalgia Impact Questionnaire score in comparison to those used the Fibromyalgia self-help course [13]. In another study on the effectiveness of physical training versus education in FM patients, *Burckhardt et al.* reported a significant impact on self-efficacy and overall quality of life. Patients who were enrolled in one or both treatments had significant decrease in physical dysfunction, pain and tenderness [14]. In a study that included 152 women with FM who were enrolled in a self-management education program, a supervised aerobic exercise program, or a combination of both for 12 weeks, *King et al.* reported an increase in walking distance post-test in the group enrolled in the supervised exercise program, and improvement in the ability to cope with symptoms of FM in those enrolled in both programs [15]. *Sosa-Reina et al.* noted that combining different types of exercises such as muscle strengthening, aerobic and stretching was most effective in improving the global well-being of patients [16]. Their findings are in accord with other researchers who also reported that mixed exercise training protocols that combine two or more types of exercises including resistance, flexibility and aerobics, improve health-related quality of life and physical well being and function, although the strength of evidence supporting this relation was only moderate [17].

Aerobic exercises also help in treating the mental well-being of affected patients. Increasing the level of activity stimulates the release of endorphins which act as an anti-depressant. In a systematic review and meta-analysis of randomised controlled trials on the effectiveness of aerobic exercise in FM, 78.1% of the participants reported that aerobic exercises reduced fatigue and pain, and helped alleviate depression. Moreover, there was marked improvement in fitness and various health-related quality of life domains. The authors recommended exercises of moderate intensity 2–3 times per week for 4 weeks [18]. In another systematic review on the effectiveness of therapeutic exercise in FM, *Sosa-Reina et al.* reported reduction in pain, depression and improvement in the physical and mental components of health-related quality of life following treatment [16].

Diet

Many FM patients exhibit symptoms similar to those reported by patients with diet-related gastro-intestinal (GI) disorders. A common example is gluten sensitivity which often results in symptoms that overlap with those of FM such as nausea, bloating, dyspepsia and body fatigue. The commonalty in symptoms between these two conditions has fostered research looking at the impact of dietary changes on the clinical course of FM. *Bjorklund et al.* advocated optimising the bioavailability of essential nutrients to reduce pain in affected patients. Their recommendation was based on the premise that muscle pain in FM could be due to an imbalance in nutrients such as amino acids, magnesium and metals which might result in disturbance in the inhibitory mechanisms [19]. *Pagliai et al.* reviewed the role of dietary supplements in FM and noted that some clinical trials advocated the intake of pro-biotics, iron and magnesium. The authors also highlighted the benefits of vegetarian diet among other diet modifications to improve the symptoms of FM [20]. In a review on the effect of diet on FM, *Metyas et al.* noted that dietary modifications, among others life style changes such as exercise, are paramount in improving the clinical course of the disease [21]. In another review that included four clinical trials and two cohort studies, *Nadal-Nicolas et al.* reported significant improvement in quality of life and general health of FM patients following a vegan diet [22]. In a study that included 75 patients, 40 of whom had adhered to a gluten-free diet for 6 months, *Slim et al.* reported a significant reduction in gluten sensitivity symptoms and improvement in FM. Notably, the gluten- free diet was not superior to the hypocaloric diet [23]. *Schrepf et al.* investigated the impact of weight loss on pain and other symptoms in FM patients and found significant improvement following 12–16-weeks of caloric restriction. There was also a decrease in severity of depression and numerous somatic symptoms after weight reduction. The authors attributed the improvement in spatial distribution of pain and comorbid symptoms to an increase in regulatory cytokine interleukin-10 [24].

Acupuncture

Acupuncture is a sensory stimulation therapy commonly used for the treatment of various chronic pain conditions [7]. Treatment outcome varies with the type of technique, traditional versus non-traditional (electroacupuncture, dry needling), number of needles used, duration of needle insertion, and patient-related factors such as mental well-being. The beneficial role of acupuncture as a non-conventional treatment option in FM has been reported by many authors. *Valera-Calero et al.*

conducted a systematic review of the literature on the efficacy of dry needling and acupuncture in FM patients and noted improvement in pain, fatigue and mental well-being of patients with both techniques [25]. In another systematic review that included 12 randomized controlled study (RCT), *Xin-Chang Zhang et al.* reported the superiority of acupuncture over sham puncture. Acupuncture was successful in reducing pain and improving patient quality of life on short and long-term follow up [26]. *Di Carlo et al.* investigated the efficacy of 8-week acupuncture treatment in patients with Fibromyalgia Impact Questionnaire (FIQ-R) above or equal to 39 and Patient Health Questionnaire 15-item above or equal to five despite medical therapy. There was a significant improvement in disease severity, pain catastrophizing and mostly in neuropathic pain features which were hard to control using drug therapy. The authors advocated the addition of acupuncture to the comprehensive approach in managing FM patients, particularly those who are refractory to traditional treatment modalities [27].

Pharmacological Treatment of Fibromyalgia

Clinical trials over the years investigated several medications using measures of quality of life, pain intensity and mental distress [28–41]. Currently, there are only three FDA-approved medications for the treatment of Fibromyalgia: duloxetine, pregabalin and milnacipran [42].

Duloxetine

Duloxetine is a serotonin-norepinephrine reuptake inhibitor (SNRI) that targets both the serotonin transporter (SERT) and norepinephrine transporter (NET), which share structural similarities, including a 12-transmembrane domain that facilitates neurotransmitter binding. Duloxetine exhibits balanced inhibition of both SERT and NET with more affinity for SERT. This pharmacological class does not possess strong antihistamine, α-adrenergic blocking, or anticholinergic properties, which contributes to its improved tolerability [43]. Common side effects of duloxetine included nausea, headache, dry mouth, constipation, somnolence, decreased appetite, hyperhidrosis, and tremor [44].

Multiple high-quality studies have been conducted over the years to investigate the role of duloxetine in Fibromyalgia management. In 2004, Arnold et al. conducted a randomized clinical trial on 207 FM patients to assess the efficacy and safety of duloxetine. The authors found that patients taking duloxetine at doses of 60 and 120 mg/day had more improvement in the overall Fibromyalgia Impact Questionnaire (FIQ) score ($P = 0.027$), Patient Global Impression of Change (PGIC) ($P = 0.033$), and pain intensity assessed using the Brief Pain Inventory (BPI) ($P = 0.008$) in comparison to the placebo group. The authors attributed patients' improvements to duloxetine's direct effect on pain, and its moderate impact on anxiety and depression [45]. In a study that included 38 Fibromyalgia patients, Russell et al. found that duloxetine at doses of 60 mg/day and 120 mg/day had significant improvement in the Brief Pain Inventory (BPI) average pain severity score and the Patient Global Impressions of Improvement (PGI-I) score, among other outcome measures [17]. In 2011, Arnold et al. investigated the long-term effect of duloxetine in patients with FM. The study included 530 patients randomized to duloxetine 60–120 mg/day (N = 263) or placebo (N = 267). Results showed significant improvement in ratings on all Multidimensional Fatigue Inventory (MFI) scales, Brief Pain Inventory (BPI) pain, anxiety, depression, and stiffness compared to placebo at week 12 ($P < 0.05$). Improvements were maintained in the duloxetine group at week 24. However, improvements in sleep quality were significant only at weeks 4 and 8 [46].

Milnacipran

Milnacipran, a SNRI with activity similar to that of duloxetine, has been studied in numerous clinical trials as a treatment for of FM symptoms. In 2004, Vitton et al. conducted a randomized clinical trial to assess the efficacy of milnacipran (200 mg/day) in managing 125 FM patients. The authors reported significant improvement in PGIC score with milnacipran compared with the placebo group ($P = 0.003$). Moreover, 37% of patients treated with milnacipran reported a 50% reduction in pain intensity in comparison with 14% in the placebo group ($P < 0.05$) [47]. In 2008, Mease et al. conducted a randomized placebo controlled clinical trial to compare the efficacy and safety of milnacipran at 100 mg/day and 200 mg/day in a cohort of 888 FM patients. There was significant improvement in the PGIC score with both doses in comparison to placebo (milnacipran 200 mg/day, $p < 0.001$; milnacipran 100 mg/day, $p = 0.009$). On the short form quality of life assessment (SF-36), both doses of milnacipran showed improvement in the SF-36 domains of bodily pain (milnacipran 200 mg/day, $p = 0.004$; milnacipran 100 mg/day, $p = 0.043$) and mental health (milnacipran 200 mg/day, $p = 0.015$; milnacipran 100 mg/day, $p = 0.007$) compared to the placebo group [48]. However, a more recent study by Pickering et al. that included 54 women with FM, found no significant difference between milnacipran 100 mg/day and placebo ($P = 0.55$) in regards to pain severity at 1-month post-treatment [49].

Pregabalin

Pregabalin, referred to as "gabapentinoid", is an amino acid-like compound that is used to manage focal seizures and a range of non-epileptic conditions, including neuropathic pain, restless leg syndrome, and anxiety disorders. Although pregabalin is structurally similar to Gamma-Aminobutyric Acid (GABA), it does not exert its effects through GABA receptors or other GABA-mediated pathways. Instead, it binds strongly to α2δ, a protein that acts as an auxiliary subunit of voltage-gated calcium channels. Pregabalin is typically well tolerated, with the most frequently reported side effects being drowsiness, dizziness, ataxia, headache and tremor. These effects are usually most pronounced at the start of treatment and often diminish with continued use. Additionally, pregabalin may lead to weight gain and peripheral edema [43].

Pregabalin has been investigated as a treatment for Fibromyalgia due to preliminary evidence suggesting that the condition may be linked to an overabundance of excitatory neurotransmitters. By reducing calcium influx, pregabalin decreases the release of excitatory neurotransmitters, including substance P, glutamate, and norepinephrine [50]. In 2008, Arnold et al. conducted a placebo-controlled clinical trial to evaluate the effectiveness and safety of pregabalin in the treatment of Fibromyalgia. The study included 750 patients diagnosed with Fibromyalgia according to the ACR criteria who were assigned randomly to receive either pregabalin at doses of 300 mg/day, 450 mg/day, or 600 mg/day, or a placebo. The authors found that pregabalin was significantly more effective than placebo in reducing pain, with greater improvements seen across all pregabalin doses ($P < 0.001$ for all doses). Pregabalin also led to significant improvements in FIQ total scores for the 450 mg/day and 600 mg/day doses ($P = 0.004$ and $P = 0.003$, respectively). All pregabalin groups showed significant improvement in sleep quality compared to placebo [50]. In 2008, Crofford et al. led a randomized, double-blind trial to evaluate the long-term efficacy of pregabalin in managing Fibromyalgia pain. The study included 1059 FM patients, 279 of whom were randomized to pregabalin. The primary outcome was the time to loss of therapeutic response (LTR), defined as less than a 30% reduction in pain or worsening FM. Pregabalin showed a significantly longer time to LTR compared to placebo, with 61% of placebo patients reaching LTR by the end of the trial versus 32% of pregabalin patients ($P < 0.001$). Overall, pregabalin demonstrated sustained effectiveness in reducing FM pain for those who responded to the treatment [51].

In 2019, Bidari et al. compared the efficacy of duloxetine and pregabalin in managing pain and depression in patients with FM using the Widespread Pain Index (WPI) and the Beck Depression Inventory (BDI). The study included 99 patients with 60 patients randomized to duloxetine and 39 patients randomized to pregabalin. The authors reported a significant difference in WPI scores between the two groups ($P = 0.034$). However, there was no significant difference in BDI scores between the two groups ($P = 0.53$) [52]. In 2020, Fatah and Elnemr compared the efficacy and tolerability of pregabalin monotherapy and the association of pregabalin and milnacipran in a study that included 58 female FM patients, using the FIQ and VAS for pain severity as primary outcome measures. At follow-up, there was a statistically significant difference in the VAS and FIQ scores in both groups ($P < 0.001$), indicating that using both of those medications has no advantage over pregabalin monotherapy [53].

Other Medications

Amitriptyline Amitriptyline is the most investigated tricyclic antidepressant (TCA) in the treatment of FM [29]. This pharmacological class inhibits the reuptake of serotonin and norepinephrine in the spinal neurons resulting in increase in their levels. By modulating both serotonin and norepinephrine pathways, TCAs influence descending pain inhibitory pathways in the central nervous system. They are considered effective for certain chronic pain conditions such as FM despite their side effect profile [43]. In a systematic review by Nishishinya et al., the authors analyzed ten randomized controlled trials on the efficacy and safety of amitriptyline in Fibromyalgia. Seven studies employed the American College of Rheumatology (ACR) diagnostic criteria [54], while three earlier studies used either the Smythe or Yunus criteria [55, 56]. A total of 615 patients were evaluated following treatment with amitriptyline hydrochloride administered at doses of 25 mg or 50 mg daily. Based on a review of six trials, 25 mg daily dose for 6–8 weeks provided statistically significant improvements in pain, sleep disturbances, fatigue, and global assessments by both patients and physicians at 6–8 weeks. However, these benefits diminished by 12 weeks. Based on other trials, 50 mg daily dose, showed no significant therapeutic benefit compared to placebo, and that dose-response discrepancy was not attributed to adverse effects or dropout rates. Common adverse effects included somnolence, dry mouth, gastrointestinal symptoms, and weight gain [57].

Fluoxetine Fluoxetine is a selective serotonin reuptake inhibitor (SSRI) that specifically targets serotonin transporters (SERT). SSRIs inhibit SERT by allosterically binding to a site distinct from the serotonin-binding site, reducing SERT activity by approximately 80% at therapeutic doses resulting in an increase in serotonin concentration. Unlike tricyclic antidepressants and serotonin-norepinephrine reuptake inhibitors, SSRIs have minimal effects on β-adrenoceptors and the norepinephrine transporter (NET) [43]. While SSRIs generally are tolerated better than tricyclic antidepressants (TCAs) due to fewer anticholinergic side effects, they have been shown to be less effective than TCAs in managing Fibromyalgia-related pain [58]. Based on the hypothesis that modulating serotonin levels with SSRIs might be more effective than targeting norepinephrine levels for alleviating certain Fibromyalgia symptoms [59], the use of Fluoxetine has expanded to include FM [60]. Since its first description in 1989, several randomized controlled trials (RCTs) have evaluated SSRIs in comparison to placebo and amitriptyline. In 1994, Wolfe et al. conducted a study comparing oral fluoxetine 20 mg daily with placebo in 42 women with Fibromyalgia over 6 weeks. Apart from a decrease in self-reported anxiety at 3 weeks, there were no statistically significant differences between the groups in terms of depression, anxiety, fatigue, pain, tender point scores or counts, or sleep quality. However, within the fluoxetine group, depressive symptoms measured by the Beck Depression Inventory (BDI) and Arthritis Impact Measurement Scale (AIMS) showed significant improvement from baseline at week 6 ($P = 0.04$ and $P = 0.03$, respectively) [61]. In 1996, Goldenberg et al. conducted a crossover trial comparing amitriptyline hydrochloride 25 mg daily, fluoxetine 20 mg daily, a combination of both medications, and placebo. The trial included 31 patients with Fibromyalgia aged 18–60 years. Each treatment or placebo was administered for 6 weeks, separated by 2-week washout periods. Both amitriptyline and fluoxetine significantly improved FIQ and visual analog scale (VAS) scores for pain, global well-being, and sleep disturbances. The combination therapy yielded greater improvements in those symptoms than either drug alone. The enhanced efficacy with combination therapy was hypothesized to result from increased amitriptyline concentrations due to fluoxetine's inhibition of cytochrome P-450 2D6 [57, 62].

Cyclobenzaprine Cyclobenzaprine is a muscle relaxant, structurally similar to TCAs and has a distinct pharmacological profile due to its prominent antimuscarinic effects [43]. Cyclobenzaprine is one of the most thoroughly investigated drugs in the treatment of Fibromyalgia, and several studies have been conducted to evaluate its efficacy in treating this condition [63]. Cyclobenzaprine has been studied in dosages ranging from 10 to 40 mg/day, with one trial investigating very low doses (1–4 mg/day) [64]. Among the three trials comparing it to a placebo [64–66], two reported significant improvements in sleep disturbances [65, 66], and two showed greater pain relief with cyclobenzaprine than placebo [64, 65]. However, all trials found no effect on fatigue, and only one placebo-controlled study showed a modest positive effect on depressive symptoms, which was not clinically significant [64]. In a study conducted in 2023, Lederman et al. conducted the RELIEF trial, a double-blind, randomized, placebo-controlled study, to assess the efficacy and safety of TNX-102 SL, a sublingual formulation of cyclobenzaprine, in treating Fibromyalgia (FM) pain. A total of 503 patients was enrolled, with 248 receiving TNX-102 SL. The primary outcome, a reduction in daily pain scores at week 14, showed a significant improvement with TNX-102 SL. Secondary outcomes including Fibromyalgia Impact Questionnaire Revised (FIQR), PROMIS Sleep Disturbance and Fatigue scores also improved in the TNX-102 SL group in comparison to the placebo group. The authors concluded that TNX-102 SL was tolerated well, reduced pain significantly and was safe for patients with FM with the most common side effects being oral hypoesthesia, oral paresthesia, and taste abnormalities [67].

Tramadol Tramadol is considered an atypical analgesic as it acts both as a weak agonist at μ-opioid receptors and as an inhibitor of serotonin and norepinephrine reuptake. Intravenous tramadol has been shown to reduce pain in Fibromyalgia patients [68]. Oral tramadol has been studied for Fibromyalgia treatment both alone and in combination with paracetamol. In a short-term placebo-controlled study, oral tramadol led to a significantly longer time before patients discontinued treatment due to inadequate pain relief compared to placebo [69]. When combined with paracetamol, it helped reduce pain, improve physical functioning, and lower the total Fibromyalgia Impact Questionnaire (FIQ) score [70]. However, oral tramadol was linked to a 19% dropout rate in both studies due to adverse events. The use of tramadol for Fibromyalgia treatment is recommended in various clinical guidelines, including those from European League Against Rheumatism (EULAR), and from several authors in Germany, Spain and Canada [71–74].

All previous clinical trials have proven that there is no gold standard treatment to manage symptoms of Fibromyalgia. In fact, managing Fibromyalgia presents a prominent challenge due to various factors. The multifaceted nature of this condition and the lack of understanding of its pathophysiology makes it difficult to pinpoint a single treatment approach resulting in the heterogeneity of treatment recommendations [75]. Another factor is the non-adherence of patients to the treatments. A review by Junior et al. reported that adherence to Fibromyalgia treatment often is hindered by noncompliance with prescriptions, particularly with regards to dose reduction or treatment discontinuation. The main contributing factor to non-adherence is thought to be the complex nature of the syndrome itself and the significant adverse effects associated with the medications prescribed. However, other factors such as the patient's age, pain intensity, polypharmacy, doctor-patient relationship, and socioeconomic conditions also contribute to the problem [76].

While significant progress has been made in understanding and managing Fibromyalgia, there still is a critical need for future research to address the gaps in treatment efficacy and personalization. Larger and more recent clinical trials are essential to validate the effectiveness of existing therapies and to explore novel approaches. Studies combining multiple medications could provide insights into synergistic effects and optimize treatment protocols. Additionally, thoroughly investigating combining pharmacological and non-pharmacological interventions trials could offer a more comprehensive understanding of multimodal approaches to managing Fibromyalgia symptoms. Furthermore, the emerging field of pharmacogenomics holds great promise in tailoring treatments to individual genetic profiles, potentially improving outcomes and reducing adverse effects. Advancing these areas of research will be vital in developing more effective, patient-centered strategies for Fibromyalgia care.

Treatment-Induced Dysphonia in Patients with FM

There are no studies in the literature on treatment-induced dysphonia in patients with FM However there are many on voice changes secondary to xerostomia, a rare side effect of the medications commonly used for the treatment of FM (Table 15.1). The prevalence of xerostomia in patient treated with duloxetine, milnacipran or pregabalin, ranges between 5% and 15% [77–79]. Xerostomia may be associated with laryngitis, gastroesophageal reflux, and throat dryness, and it can worsen voice quality of affected patients.

Xerostomia is defined as dryness in the mouth that can be due to many causes such as autoimmune diseases, radiation therapy for the head and neck malignancies, and the intake of various classes of medications [80]. Xerostomia can impact voice particularly because the dryness often extend the laryngeal mucosal surface. Superficial dehydration of the vocal folds, whether caused by systemic dehydration or medications, results in impaired oscillation that leads to an increase in vocal effort and an increase in the phonatory threshold pressure, that is the pressure needed to set the vocal folds into vibration. With increase in PTP and the collision

Table 15.1 Overview of Fibromyalgia Medications, typical dosages and potential side effects

Medication	Dose	Side effects
Duloxetine [44]	30 mg once daily for 1 week, then increase to 60 mg once daily as tolerated	Laryngitis, xerostomia, cough, nasopharyngitis, nausea
Milnacipran [49]	12.5 mg once daily on day 1, then 12.5 mg twice daily on days 2 to 3, 25 mg twice daily on days 4 to 7, then to usual dosage of 50 mg twice daily thereafter	Reflux, xerostomia, nausea
	Dose may be increased to 100 mg twice daily, based on individual response	
Pregabalin [50]	75 mg twice daily; may increase to 150 mg twice daily within 1 week based on response and tolerability; maximum dose: 450 mg/day	Xerostomia, nasopharyngitis, pharyngolaryngeal pain, nausea
Amitriptyline [57]	10 mg once daily, 1 to 3 h before bedtime; gradually increase dose based on response and tolerability in 5 to 10 mg increments at intervals of ≥2 weeks up to 75 mg/day	Xerostomia, nausea
Fluoxetine [61]	20 mg once daily; may increase dose based on response and tolerability in 10 to 20 mg increments at ≥2-week intervals up to 80 mg/day	Xerostomia, pharyngitis, laryngeal edema, nausea
Cyclobenzaprine [66]	5 to 10 mg once daily before bedtime; may gradually titrate as needed and tolerated up to 10 to 40 mg daily in 1 to 3 divided doses	Xerostomia, pharyngitis, nausea
Tramadol [70]	25 to 50 mg every 6 h as needed. The dose may be increased as needed and tolerated to 50 to 100 mg every 4 to 6 h (maximum: 400 mg/day)	Xerostomia, cough, nasopharyngitis, pharyngitis, nausea

forces between the vocal folds during phonation, there is higher risk for development of functional and structural voice disorders [81–83]. *Grinstein-Koren* investigated the voice characteristics of 24 women diagnosed with dry mouth and noted higher mean Voice Handicap Index-10 (VHI-10) score and higher ratings of the auditory perceptual evaluation in comparison to controls. The subjective evaluation was substantiated objectively. Acoustic analysis showed lower fundamental frequency and higher jitter in patients with dry mouth in comparison to those with no dry mouth [84]. *Roh et al.* examined voice function in 10 men with drug-induced xerostomia and noted a significant increase in phonation threshold pressure and vocal effort in comparison to controls who had no xerostomia. There was also a high correlation between the voice changes and the decrease in salivary flow [85].

The correlation between xerostomia and dysphonia is supported further by the numerous reports on the link between hyposalivation and hoarseness in patients with Sjogren's syndrome (SS) and in patients treated with radiation therapy for head and neck cancer. *Pierce et al.* investigated the prevalence of voice disorders in 101 patients with SS using a questionnaire and noted a current voice disorder in 59.4% of the cases. Moreover, there was a significant association between throat dryness and severity of disease. The authors highlighted the need to address the voice complaint in the evaluation and management of affected patients [86]. *Salturk et al.* reported a significant difference in vocal fold smoothness and glottic closure of women with SS in comparison to healthy controls. The laryngeal video-stroboscopic findings were associated with a higher VHI-10 score and self-perceived hoarseness [87]. *Roh et al.* reported voice dysfunction and abnormal laryngeal findings on stroboscopy in patients who received wide-field irradiation for the head and neck. The authors ascribed their findings to the significant decrease in salivary flow and stressed the need to take preventive measures in patients receiving wide-field radiotherapy to head and neck cancer [88]. *Mathew et al.* investigated changes in swallowing and laryngeal function in 33 patients with laryngo-pharyngeal malignancies who underwent radiotherapy ± chemotherapy and noted an increase in laryngeal edema associated with roughness and a decrease in the mean fundamental frequency 3–6 months following treatment. The authors also reported a significant increase in the prevalence of dysphagia by 15.1% at 6 months following treatment [89]. Similar upper airway conditions and related voice dysfunction occur commonly as a result of side effects of medications used routinely to treat FM; and physicians should counsel patients (especially professional voice users) about the risk of dysphonia prior to treatment and should select a regimen that produces the least xerostomia for each individual.

Another common side effect of the medications used for the treatment of FM that may impact voice is nausea [77–79]. Nausea is defined as" a symptom precursor to the act of vomiting" and is considered by many as a warning for possible body intoxication [90]. The pathophysiology of nausea is very complex and encompasses disturbance in the central and autonomic nervous systems often leading to gastric dysrhythmias. The dysfunction in the myoelectric activity of the stomach frequently is associated with vomiting and possible purging. Both purging and vomiting behaviors have been associated with a higher prevalence of voice disorders. In a study on the relation between voice disorders and eating disorders. *Lawrence et al.* noted that purging was a risk factor for dysphonia. Almost one out of five patients in their study group had voice disorders, almost double the rate reported in the normal population [91]. The authors attributed voice problems to the physiological consequences of purging, such as gastro-esophageal reflux disease. Reflux disease is a known risk factor for dysphonia and has been associated with structural and functional voice disorders. The acidic and non-acidic refluxate contents of the stomach damage the mucosal lining of the larynx resulting in inflammatory changes such as edema and in mass formation [92], as well as in impaired defense mechanism and impaired healing from trauma.

Another explanation for the increased risk for voice disorders in patients with nausea is malnutrition. Malnutrition and emaciation can lead to atrophic changes in the vocal folds and derangement in the extracellular matrix constituents [93, 94]. This hypothesis can be extrapolated from numerous studies showing that weight loss results in atrophy of the vocal folds and compensatory hyperfunctional voice disorders [95]. Nausea also may lead to decrease in water intake resulting to in systemic dehydration. Dehydration increases the phonation threshold pressure and vocal effort. Patients subjected to local dehydration following inhalation of dry desiccated air, or to systemic dehydration following religious rituals or the intake of drugs suffer from voice fatigue and increase in phonatory effort. Nausea also may decrease the ability of the speaker to use his or her abdominal muscles for breathing support and control. Although there are no studies on nausea and diminished contraction of the trunk muscles, singers and speakers who rely heavily on abdominal, thoracic and back muscle efficient contraction are likely to have phonation impaired by restrictions in muscle use necessitated by nausea.

References

1. Aman MM, Jason Yong R, Kaye AD, Urman RD. Evidence-based non-pharmacological therapies for fibromyalgia. Curr Pain Headache Rep. 2018;22(5):33.
2. García-Ríos MC, Navarro-Ledesma S, Tapia-Haro RM, Toledano-Moreno S, Casas-Barragán A, Correa-Rodríguez M, Aguilar-Ferrándiz ME. Effectiveness of health education in patients with fibromyalgia: a systematic review. Eur J Phys Rehabil Med. 2019;55(2):301–13.
3. Macfarlane GJ, Kronisch C, Dean LE, et al. EULAR revised recommendations for the management of fibromyalgia. Ann Rheum Dis. 2017;76(2):318–28.
4. Bernardy K, Füber N, Klose P, Häuser W. Efficacy of hypnosis/guided imagery in fibromyalgia syndrome—a systematic review and meta-analysis of controlled trials. BMC Musculoskelet Disord. 2011;12:133.
5. Glombiewski JA, Sawyer AT, Gutermann J, Koenig K, Rief W, Hofmann SG. Psychological treatments for fibromyalgia: a meta-analysis. Pain. 2010;151(2):280–95.
6. Falcão DM, Sales L, Leite JR, Feldman D, Valim V, Natour J. Cognitive behavioral therapy for the treatment of fibromyalgia syndrome: a randomized controlled trial. J Musculoskeletal Pain. 2008;16(3):133–40.
7. Adler-Neal AL, Zeidan F. Mindfulness meditation for fibromyalgia: mechanistic and clinical considerations. Curr Rheumatol Rep. 2017;19(9):59.
8. Meng S, Cao C, Zhang M, Dong J, Lu M. Mindfulness meditation for fibromyalgia syndrome: a systematic review and meta-analysis. Pain Physician. 2024;27(8):479–94.
9. Cash E, Salmon P, Weissbecker I, Rebholz WN, Bayley-Veloso R, Zimmaro LA, Floyd A, Dedert E, Sephton SE. Mindfulness meditation alleviates fibromyalgia symptoms in women: results of a randomized clinical trial. Ann Behav Med. 2015;49(3):319–30.
10. Shonin E, Van Gordon W. Managers' experiences of meditation awareness training. Mindfulness. 2015;6:899–909.
11. Van Gordon W, Shonin E, Dunn TJ, Garcia-Campayo J, Griffiths MD. Meditation awareness training for the treatment of fibromyalgia syndrome: a randomized controlled trial. Br J Health Psychol. 2017;22(1):186–206.
12. Izquierdo-Alventosa R, Inglés M, Cortés-Amador S, et al. Low-intensity physical exercise improves pain catastrophizing and other psychological and physical aspects in women with fibromyalgia: a randomized controlled trial. Int J Environ Res Public Health. 2020;17(10):3634.
13. Rooks DS, Gautam S, Romeling M, Cross ML, Stratigakis D, Evans B, Goldenberg DL, Iversen MD, Katz JN. Group exercise, education, and combination self-management in women with fibromyalgia: a randomized trial. Arch Intern Med. 2007;167(20):2192–200.
14. Burckhardt CS, Bjelle A. Education programmes for fibromyalgia patients: description and evaluation. Baillieres Clin Rheumatol. 1994;8(4):935–55.
15. King SJ, Wessel J, Bhambhani Y, Sholter D, Maksymowych W. The effects of exercise and education, individually or combined, in women with fibromyalgia. J Rheumatol. 2002;29(12):2620–7.

16. Sosa-Reina MD, Nunez-Nagy S, Gallego-Izquierdo T, Pecos-Martín D, Monserrat J, Álvarez-Mon M. Effectiveness of therapeutic exercise in fibromyalgia syndrome: a systematic review and meta-analysis of randomized clinical trials. Biomed Res Int. 2017;2017:2356346.
17. Bidonde J, Busch AJ, Schachter CL, Webber SC, Musselman KE, Overend TJ, Góes SM, Dal Bello-Haas V, Boden C. Mixed exercise training for adults with fibromyalgia. Cochrane Database Syst Rev. 2019;5(5):CD013340.
18. Häuser W, Klose P, Langhorst J, Moradi B, Steinbach M, Schiltenwolf M, Busch A. Efficacy of different types of aerobic exercise in fibromyalgia syndrome: a systematic review and meta-analysis of randomised controlled trials. Arthritis Res Ther. 2010;12:1–4.
19. Bjørklund G, Dadar M, Chirumbolo S, Aaseth J. Fibromyalgia and nutrition: therapeutic possibilities? Biomed Pharmacother. 2018;103:531–8.
20. Pagliai G, Giangrandi I, Dinu M, Sofi F, Colombini B. Nutritional interventions in the management of fibromyalgia syndrome. Nutrients. 2020;12(9):2525.
21. Metyas C, Aung TT, Cheung J, Joseph M, Ballester AM, Metyas S. Diet and lifestyle modifications for fibromyalgia. Curr Rheumatol Rev. 2024;20(4):405–13.
22. Nadal-Nicolás Y, Miralles-Amorós L, Martínez-Olcina M, Sánchez-Ortega M, Mora J, Martínez-Rodríguez A. Vegetarian and vegan diet in fibromyalgia: a systematic review. Int J Environ Res Public Health. 2021;18(9):4955.
23. Slim M, Calandre EP, Garcia-Leiva JM, et al. The effects of a gluten-free diet versus a hypocaloric diet among patients with fibromyalgia experiencing gluten sensitivity-like symptoms: a pilot, open-label randomized clinical trial. J Clin Gastroenterol. 2017;51(6):500–7.
24. Schrepf A, Harte SE, Miller N, Fowler C, Nay C, Williams DA, Clauw DJ, Rothberg A. Improvement in the spatial distribution of pain, somatic symptoms, and depression after a weight loss intervention. J Pain. 2017;18(12):1542–50.
25. Valera-Calero JA, Fernández-de-Las-Peñas C, Navarro-Santana MJ, Plaza-Manzano G. Efficacy of dry needling and acupuncture in patients with fibromyalgia: a systematic review and meta-analysis. Int J Environ Res Public Health. 2022;19(16):9904.
26. Zhang XC, Chen H, Xu WT, Song YY, Gu YH, Ni GX. Acupuncture therapy for fibromyalgia: a systematic review and meta-analysis of randomized controlled trials. J Pain Res. 2019;12:527–42.
27. Di Carlo M, Beci G, Salaffi F. Acupuncture for fibromyalgia: an open-label pragmatic study on effects on disease severity, neuropathic pain features, and pain catastrophizing. Evid Based Complement Alternat Med. 2020;2020:9869250.
28. Arnold LM, Clauw DJ. Challenges of implementing fibromyalgia treatment guidelines in current clinical practice. Postgrad Med. 2017;129(7):709–14.
29. Traynor LM, Thiessen CN, Traynor AP. Pharmacotherapy of fibromyalgia. Am J Health Syst Pharm. 2011;68(14):1307–19.
30. Myles PS, Troedel S, Boquest M, et al. The pain visual analog scale; is it linear or nonlinear? Anesth Analg. 1999;89:1517–20.
31. Keller S, Bann CM, Dodd SL, et al. Validity of the brief pain inventory for use in documenting the outcomes of patients with noncancer pain. Clin J Pain. 2004;20:309–18.
32. Melzack R. The McGill Pain Questionnaire: major properties and scoring methods. Pain. 1975;1:277–99.
33. Bennett R. The Fibromyalgia Impact Questionnaire (FIQ): a review of its development, current version, operating characteristics and uses. Clin Exp Rheumatol. 2005;23(suppl 39):S154–62.
34. Ware JE, Sherbourne CD. The MOS 36-Item Short-Form Health Survey (SF-36): I. Conceptual framework and item selection. Med Care. 1992;30:473–83.
35. Hurst H, Bolton J. Assessing the clinical significance of change scores recorded on subjective outcome measures. J Manip Physiol Ther. 2004;27:26–35.
36. Guy W. Clinical global impressions. In: ECDEU assessment manual for psycho- pharmacology. Rockville: Department of Health, Education, and Welfare; 1976. p. 217–22.
37. Hays RD, Stewart AL. Sleep measures. In: Stewart AL, Ware JE, editors. Measuring functioning and well-being: the Medical Outcomes Study approach. Durham: Duke University Press; 1992. p. 235–359.

38. Buysse DJ, Reynolds CF, Monk TH, et al. The Pittsburgh Sleep Quality Index (PSQI): a new instrument for psychiatric research and practice. Psychiatry Res. 1989;28:193–213.
39. Meenan RF, Gertman PM, Mason JH. Measuring health status in arthritis: the Arthritis Impact Measurement Scales. Arthritis Rheum. 1980;23:146–52.
40. Beck AT, Ward C, Mendelson M. Beck depression inventory (BDI). Arch Gen Psychiatry. 1961;4:561–71.
41. Smets EM, Garssen B, Bonke B, et al. The multidimensional fatigue inventory (MFI) psychometric qualities of an instrument to assess fatigue. J Psychosom Res. 1995;39:315–25.
42. Tzadok R, Ablin JN. Current and emerging pharmacotherapy for fibromyalgia. Pain Res Manag. 2020;2020:6541798.
43. Katzung BG, editor. Basic and clinical pharmacology. 14th ed. San Francisco: Lange Medical; 2018.
44. Russell IJ, Mease PJ, Smith TR, et al. Efficacy and safety of duloxetine for treatment of fibromyalgia in patients with or without major depressive disorder: results from a 6-month, randomized, double-blind, placebo-controlled, fixed- dose trial. Pain. 2008;136:432–44.
45. Arnold LM, Lu Y, Crofford LJ, et al. A double-blind, multicenter trial comparing duloxetine with placebo in the treatment of fibromyalgia patients with or without major depressive disorder. Arthritis Rheum. 2004;50:2974–84.
46. Arnold LM, Wang F, Ahl J, Gaynor PJ, Wohlreich MM. Improvement in multiple dimensions of fatigue in patients with fibromyalgia treated with duloxetine: secondary analysis of a randomized, placebo-controlled trial. Arthritis Res Ther. 2011;13(3):R86.
47. Vitton O, Gendreau M, Gendreau J, et al. A double-blind placebo-controlled trial of milnacipran in the treatment of fibro- myalgia. Hum Psychopharmacol. 2004;19(suppl 1):S27–35.
48. Mease PJ, Clauw DJ, Gendreau RM, et al. The efficacy and safety of milnacipran for treatment of fibromyalgia. A randomized, double-blind, placebo-controlled trial. J Rheumatol. 2009;36:398–409.
49. Pickering G, Macian N, Delage N, Picard P, Cardot JM, Sickout-Arondo S, Giron F, Dualé C, Pereira B, Marcaillou F. Milnacipran poorly modulates pain in patients suffering from fibromyalgia: a randomized double-blind controlled study. Drug Des Devel Ther. 2018;12:2485–96.
50. Arnold LM, Russell IJ, Diri EW, et al. A 14-week, randomized, double-blinded, placebo-controlled monotherapy trial of pregabalin in patients with fibromyalgia. J Pain. 2008;9(9):792–805.
51. Crofford LJ, Mease PJ, Simpson SL, et al. Fibromyalgia Relapse Evaluation and Efficacy for Durability of Meaningful Relief (FREEDOM): a 6-month, double-blind, placebo-controlled trial with pregabalin. Pain. 2008;136:419–31.
52. Bidari A, Moazen-Zadeh E, Ghavidel-Parsa B, Rahmani S, Hosseini S, Hassankhani A. Comparing duloxetine and pregabalin for treatment of pain and depression in women with fibromyalgia: an open-label randomized clinical trial. Daru. 2019;27(1):149–58.
53. Abdel Fattah YH, Elnemr R. Efficacy of pregabalin as a monotherapy versus combined pregabalin and milnacipran in the management of fibromyalgia. Int J Rheum Dis. 2020;23(11):1474–80.
54. Wolfe F, Smythe HA, Yunus MB, Bennett RM, Bombardier C, Goldenberg DL, Tugwell P, Campbell SM, Abeles M, Clark P, et al. The American college of rheumatology 1990 criteria for the classification of fibromyalgia. Report of the multicenter criteria committee. Arthritis Rheum. 1990;33(2):160–72.
55. Smythe HA. "Fibrositis" is a disorder of pain modulation. Clin Rheum Dis. 1979;5:823–32.
56. Yunus M, Masi AT, Calabro JJ, Miller KA, Feigenbaum SL. Primary fibromyalgia (fibrositis): clinical study of 50 patients with matched normal controls. Semin Arthritis Rheum. 1981;11(1):151–71.
57. Nishishinya B, Urrutia G, Walitt B, et al. Amitriptyline in the treatment of fibromyalgia: a systematic review of its efficacy. Rheumatology. 2008;47:1741–6.
58. Geller SA. Treatment of fibrositis with fluoxetine hydrochloride (Prozac). Am J Med. 1989;87:594–5.
59. Sarzi-Puttini P, Torta R, Marinangeli F, et al. Fibromyalgia syndrome: the pharmacological treatment options. Reumatismo. 2008;60(suppl 1):50–8.

60. Goldenberg D, Mayskiy M, Mossey C, et al. A randomized, double-blind crossover trial of fluoxetine and amitriptyline in the treatment of fibromyalgia. Arthritis Rheum. 1996;39:1852–9.
61. Wolfe F, Cathey MA, Hawley DJ. A double-blind placebo controlled trial of fluoxetine in fibromyalgia. Scand J Rheumatol. 1994;23:255–9.
62. Miller LJ, Kubes KL. Serotonergic agents in the treatment of fibromyalgia syndrome. Ann Pharmacother. 2002;36:707–12.
63. Calandre EP, Rico-Villademoros F, Slim M. An update on pharmacotherapy for the treatment of fibromyalgia. Expert Opin Pharmacother. 2015;16(9):1347–68.
64. Moldofsky H, Harris HW, Archambault WT, et al. Effects of bedtime very low dose cyclobenzaprine on symptoms and sleep physiology in patients with fibromyalgia syndrome: a double-blind randomized placebo- controlled study. J Rheumatol. 2011;38:2653–63.
65. Bennett RM, Gatter RA, Campbell SM, et al. A comparison of cyclobenzaprine and placebo in the management of fibrositis. A double-blind controlled study. Arthritis Rheum. 1988;31:1535–42.
66. Quimby LG, Gratwick GM, Whitney CD, et al. A randomized trial of cyclobenzaprine for the treatment of fibromyalgia. J Rheumatol Suppl. 1989;19:140–3.
67. Lederman S, Arnold LM, Vaughn B, Kelley M, Sullivan GM. Efficacy and safety of sublingual cyclobenzaprine for the treatment of fibromyalgia: results from a randomized, double-blind, placebo-controlled trial. Arthritis Care Res (Hoboken). 2023;75(11):2359–68.
68. Biasi G, Manca S, Manganelli S, et al. Tramadol in the fibromyalgia syndrome: a controlled clinical trial versus placebo. Int J Clin Pharmacol Res. 1998;18:13–9.
69. Russell IJ, Kamin M, Bennett RM, et al. Efficacy of tramadol in treatment of pain in fibromyalgia. J Clin Rheumatol. 2000;6:250–7.
70. Bennett RM, Kamin M, Karim R, et al. Tramadol and acetaminophen combination tablets in the treatment of fibromyalgia pain: a double-blind, randomized, placebo-controlled study. Am J Med. 2003;114:537–45.
71. Carville SF, Arendt-Nielsen S, Bliddal H, et al. EULAR evidence-based recommendations for the management of fibromyalgia syndrome. Ann Rheum Dis. 2008;67:536–41.
72. Hauser W, Arnold B, Eich W, et al. Management of fibromyalgia syndrome—an interdisciplinary evidence-based guideline. Ger Med Sci. 2008;6:Doc14.
73. de Miquel CA, Campayo J, Florez MT, et al. Interdisciplinary consensus document for the treatment of fibromyalgia. Actas Esp Psiquiatr. 2010;38:108–20.
74. Fitzcharles MA, Ste-Marie PA, Goldenberg DL, et al. 2012;Canadian Guidelines for the diagnosis and management of fibromyalgia syndrome: executive summary. Pain Res Manag. 2013;18:119–26.
75. Sarzi-Puttini P, Giorgi V, Marotto D, Atzeni F. Fibromyalgia: an update on clinical characteristics, aetiopathogenesis and treatment. Nat Rev Rheumatol. 2020;16(11):645–60.
76. Oliveira Júnior JO, Ramos JV. Adherence to fibromyalgia treatment: challenges and impact on the quality of life. Brazil J Pain. 2019;2:81–7.
77. UpToDate. Duloxetine: drug information. https://www.uptodate.com/contents/duloxetine-drug-information
78. UpToDate. Milnacipran: drug information. https://www.uptodate.com/contents/milnacipran-drug-information
79. UpToDate. Pregabalin: drug information. https://www.uptodate.com/contents/pregabalin-drug-information
80. Millsop JW, Wang EA, Fazel N. Etiology, evaluation, and management of xerostomia. Clin Dermatol. 2017;35(5):468–76.
81. Hamdan AL, Sabra O, Rifai H, Tabri D, Hussari A. Vocal changes in patients using nasal continuous positive airway pressure. J Voice. 2008;22(5):603–6.
82. Hamdan AL, Nassar J, Dowli A, Al Zaghal Z, Sabri A. Effect of fasting on laryngopharyngeal reflux disease in male subjects. Eur Arch Otorrinolaringol. 2012;269(11):2361–6.
83. Verdolini K, Titze IR, Fennell A. Dependence of phonatory effort on hydration level. J Speech Lang Hear Res. 1994;37(5):1001–7.

84. Grinstein-Koren O, Herzog N, Amir O. Hyposalivation affecting womens' voice. J Voice. 2023;37(3):469–e19.
85. Roh JL, Kim HS, Kim AY. The effect of acute xerostomia on vocal function. Arch Otolaryngol Head Neck Surg. 2006;132(5):542–6.
86. Pierce JL, Tanner K, Merrill RM, Miller KL, Ambati BK, Kendall KA, Roy N. Voice disorders in S jögren's syndrome: prevalence and related risk factors. Laryngoscope. 2015;125(6):1385–92.
87. Saltürk Z, Özdemir E, Kumral TL, Karabacakoğlu Z, Kumral E, Yildiz HE, Mersinlioğlu G, Atar Y, Berkiten G, Yildirim G, Uyar Y. Subjective and objective voice evaluation in Sjögren's syndrome. Logoped Phoniatr Vocol. 2017;42(1):9–11.
88. Roh JL, Kim AY, Cho MJ. Xerostomia following radiotherapy of the head and neck affects vocal function. J Clin Oncol. 2005;23(13):3016–23.
89. Mathew JM, Mukherji A, Saxena SK, Vijayaraghavan N, Menon A, Sriharsha K, Rafi M. Change in dysphagia and laryngeal function after radical radiotherapy in laryngo pharyngeal malignancies—a prospective observational study. Rep Pract Oncol Radiother. 2021;26(5):655–63.
90. Singh P, Yoon SS, Kuo B. Nausea: a review of pathophysiology and therapeutics. Ther Adv Gastroenterol. 2016;9(1):98–112.
91. Lawrence T, van Mersbergen M. The relation between eating disorders and voice disorders. J Voice. 2021;35(5):753–64.
92. Lechien JR, Hamdan AL, Saussez S. Laryngopharyngeal reflux and benign lesions of the vocal folds. Eur Arch Otorrinolaringol. 2019;276:277–8.
93. Maciejewska B, Rajewska-Rager A, Maciejewska-Szaniec Z, Michalak M, Rajewski A, Wiskirska-Woźnica B. The assessment of the impact of anorexia nervosa on the vocal apparatus in adolescent girls—a preliminary report. Int J Pediatr Otorhinolaryngol. 2016;85:141–7.
94. Branski RC, Verdolini K, Sandulache V, Rosen CA, Hebda PA. Vocal fold wound healing: a review for clinicians. J Voice. 2006;20(3):432–42.
95. Kosztyła-Hojna B. The evaluation of voice and aerodynamic activity of larynx in patients with vocal cords atrophy. Polski Merkuriusz Lekarski. 2005;18(104):151–5.

Conclusion

16

Abdul-latif Hamdan, Robert Thayer Sataloff,
and Mary J. Hawkshaw

It is important for otolaryngologists and voice care providers to know that Fibromyalgia (FM) is a systemic disorder that does not spare the phonatory apparatus. Although subtle in nature and often masked by other symptoms such as body fatigue and pain, hoarseness is a common manifestation of this debilitating syndrome that causes a large array of somatic and non-somatic complaints. Hoarseness can be the result of dysfunction in both the oscillator and power source for phonation. The decrease in musculoskeletal endurance and strength may lead to hyperfunctional compensatory muscle recruitment, voice fatigue and phonatory symptoms as a result of laryngeal muscle involvement [1, 2]. Similarly, patients may complain of dysphagia, food stuck in their throat and aspiration secondary to dysfunction in the pharyngeal muscles [3, 4]. The respiratory muscles also are affected in FM. Studies have shown that FM patients have a decrease in inspiratory and expiratory muscle activity and a decrease in chest wall compliance. The weakness in the respiratory muscles results in dyspnea and shortness of breath that compromise the ability of the patient to talk for prolonged periods of time and often lead to volume disturbance. In professional voice users with FM, both breath support and control of voice can be affected. Singers may have trouble modulating the subglottic pressure with change in voice pitch. Loss of the intricate control of diaphragm and other respiratory muscle activity may result in difficulty in sustaining a note and in transition between registers [5–8].

With our improved understanding of the pathophysiology of FM, several mechanisms to explain dysphonia in FM patients have been suggested. One of these is laryngeal muscle dysfunction secondary to poor muscle oxygenation, inflammation and degenerative changes [9, 10]. Laryngeal muscle function is deranged further by pain and the systemic imbalance in neuromodulators and neurotransmitters. Pain as a result of central sensitization and or alteration in the descending inhibitory pathways can lead to increased laryngeal muscle tension resulting in a spectrum of voice and swallowing symptoms [11, 12]. Future investigations are needed to elucidate the pathophysiology of dysphonia in FM patients.

A.-l. Hamdan et al., *Voice Disorders in Fibromyalgia*,
https://doi.org/10.1007/978-3-031-97751-0_16

Physicians and voice care providers also should beware that the impact of FM on the phonatory system is compounded by the various comorbidities of the syndrome, including gastro-intestinal disorders, rheumatologic disorders, sleep disorders and body fatigue. Gastro-intestinal disorders have a negative impact on the clinical course of FM and on its treatment outcome. Reflux disease for instance, may aggravate pain sensitivity by stimulating nociceptors in the esophagus [13]. Reflux disease also increases the risk for structural and functional voice disorders particularly in patients with laryngopharyngeal reflux [13, 14]. It has been estimated that one out of two patients with voice disorders suffer from laryngopharyngeal reflux even in the absence of symptoms of regurgitation and heartburn [15], and the percentage is probably higher. Patients with FM are more prone to have dysphonia in comparison to healthy subjects. Precautions such as dietary modifications and early treatment are recommended in FM patients with reflux and voice symptoms. Current literature lacks any study on the prevalence of laryngopharyngeal reflux in FM patients in comparison to healthy controls. Future investigations on the risk of dysphonia in FM patients with LPR versus those without LPR are warranted.

Rheumatologic diseases are also common in patients with FM, often masking the diagnosis and worsening the course of this syndrome. Although the use of serologic markers can help in differentiating between the two, the overlap in the clinical presentation and pathophysiology makes it hard to differentiate FM from many rheumatologic disorders. The laryngeal manifestations of rheumatoid arthritis, ankylosing spondylitis and other autoimmune disorders are known to otolaryngologists and voice care providers. Both soft tissues and joints in the laryngeal framework are affected leading to vocal fold submucosal masses such as rheumatoid nodules and bamboo nodes, and to impairment of vocal fold mobility secondary to inflammation and/or ankylosis of the cricoarytenoid joint [16]. When rheumatologic diseases co-exist with FM, affected patients are more likely to complain of voice and swallowing symptoms. Physicians should have a high index of suspicion in the work-up of patients with a history of rheumatologic disorder for possible FM. Future research in this field is needed to elucidate the prevalence of dysphonia in FM patients with rheumatologic disorders versus FM patients without rheumatologic disorders.

Insomnia and disturbance in sleep are also compounding factors that need to be considered in the work-up of FM patients with dysphonia. Patients with FM are known to suffer from various sleep disorders such as non-restorative sleep, upper airway resistance syndrome and obstructive sleep apnea [17–19]. The impact of these sleep disorders on voice is well known particularly in patients with chronic fatigue [20]. Several mechanisms have been suggested. A plausible one is sleep-induced autonomic nervous system dysfunction, although there are no studies substantiating this hypothesis in FM patients with sleep disturbances and history of dysphonia. A prospective study looking at the risk of dysphonia in FM patients with sleep disorders in comparison to another group without sleep disorders and to controls is warranted.

Physicians also must be attentive to the potential laryngologic side effects caused by medications used to treat FM. Research into alternative treatments with fewer side effects on voice should be encouraged.

In conclusion, decrease in the efficiency of the phonatory apparatus as a result of dysfunction in the oscillator and power source for phonation in FM patients is not only secondary to the disease itself, but also to the manifestation of other systemic diseases and of treatment. The patients' reported voice handicap and the change in voice characteristics in FM patients warrant a multi-disciplinary approach that addresses for the various comorbidities of this syndrome, and its management.

References

1. Gurbuzler L, Inanir A, Yelken K, Koc S, Eyibilen A, Uysal IO. Voice disorder in patients with fibromyalgia. Auris Nasus Larynx. 2013;40(6):554–7.
2. Hamdan AL, Hosri J, Yammine Y, Ghzayel L, Hadi J, Moussawi MA, Romanos M, Nader N, Uthman I. Voice disorders in patients with fibromyalgia: case series and review of the literature. J Voice. 2024; https://doi.org/10.1016/j.jvoice.2024.06.027.
3. Gilheaney Ó, Costello C, McTiernan K. Surveying the International prevalence and nature of eating, drinking and swallowing difficulties in adults presenting with fibromyalgia. Dysphagia. 2024;39(3):495–503.
4. Del Carmen Villaverde-Rodríguez M, Correa-Rodríguez M, Casas-Barragán A, Tapia-Haro RM, Aguilar-Ferrándiz ME. Orofacial pain and risk of dysphagia in women with fibromyalgia: a cross-sectional observational study. Am J Speech Lang Pathol. 2024;33(2):883–92.
5. Homann D, Stefanello JM, Góes SM, Leite N. Impaired functional capacity and exacerbation of pain and exertion during the 6-minute walk test in women with fibromyalgia. Rev Bras Fisioter. 2011;15(6):474–80. English, Portuguese.
6. Lurie M, Caidahl K, Johansson G, Bake B. Respiratory function in chronic primary fibromyalgia. Scand J Rehabil Med. 1990;22(3):151–5.
7. Forti M, Zamunér AR, Andrade CP, Silva E. Lung function, respiratory muscle strength, and thoracoabdominal mobility in women with fibromyalgia syndrome. Respir Care. 2016;61(10):1384–90.
8. Ozgocmen S, Cimen OB, Ardicoglu O. Relationship between chest expansion and respiratory muscle strength in patients with primary fibromyalgia. Clin Rheumatol. 2002;21:19–22.
9. Lund N, Bengtsson A, Thorborg P. Muscle tissue oxygen pressure in primary fibromyalgia. Scand J Rheumatol. 1986;15(2):165–73.
10. Bengtsson A, Henriksson KG, Larsson J. Reduced high-energy phosphate levels in the painful muscles of patients with primary fibromyalgia. Arthritis Rheum. 1986;29(7):817–21.
11. Pérez-Neri I, Sandoval H, Estêvão MD, Vasanthan LT, Alarcon-Ruiz CA, Ruszkowski J, Mathangasinghe Y, Ríos C, Pineda C. Central and peripheral mechanisms of pain in fibromyalgia: scoping review protocol. Rheumatol Int. 2023;43(4):757–62.
12. Lautenbacher S, Salinas-Ranneberg M, Niebuhr O, Kunz M. Phonetic characteristics of vocalizations during pain. Pain Rep. 2017;2(3):e597.
13. Wang JC, Sung FC, Men M, Wang KA, Lin CL, Kao CH. Bidirectional association between fibromyalgia and gastroesophageal reflux disease: two population-based retrospective cohort analysis. Pain. 2017;158(10):1971–8.
14. Gilheaney Ó, Chadwick A. The prevalence and nature of eating and swallowing problems in adults with fibromyalgia: a systematic review. Dysphagia. 2024;39(1):92–108.
15. Koufman J, Sataloff RT, Toohill R. Laryngopharyngeal reflux: consensus conference report. J Voice. 1996;10(3):215–6.

16. Hamdan AL, Sataloff RT, Hawkshaw MJ. Laryngeal manifestations of autoimmune diseases. Laryngeal Manifest Syst Dis. 2019;281:281–312.
17. Bigatti SM, Hernandez AM, Cronan TA, Rand KL. Sleep disturbances in fibromyalgia syndrome: relationship to pain and depression. Arthritis Rheum. 2008;59:961–7.
18. Çetin B, Sünbül EA, Toktaş H, Karaca M, Ulutaş Ö, Güleç H. Comparison of sleep structure in patients with fibromyalgia and healthy controls. Sleep Breath. 2020;24(4):1591–8.
19. Mutlu P, Zateri C, Zohra A, Ozerdogan O, Mirici AN. Prevalence of obstructive sleep apnea in female patients with fibromyalgia. Saudi Med J. 2020;41(7):740–5.
20. Hamdan AL, Sataloff RT, Hawkshaw MJ. Sleep, body fatigue and voice. Laryngeal Manifest Syst Dis. 2019;281:83–6.

Index

A.-l. Hamdan et al., *Voice Disorders in Fibromyalgia*,
https://doi.org/10.1007/978-3-031-97751-0

W

X

MIX
Papier aus verantwortungsvollen Quellen
Paper from responsible sources
FSC® C105338
FSC
www.fsc.org

If you have any concerns about our products,
you can contact us on
ProductSafety@springernature.com

In case Publisher is established outside the EU,
the EU authorized representative is:
Springer Nature Customer Service Center GmbH
Europaplatz 3, 69115 Heidelberg, Germany

Printed by Libri Plureos GmbH
in Hamburg, Germany